MANUAL OF
CHEMICAL
PEELS

Superficial and Medium Depth

MANUAL OF CHEMICAL PEELS

Superficial and Medium Depth

Mark G. Rubin, MD

Assistant Clinical Professor
Division of Dermatology
University of California, San Diego
San Diego, California

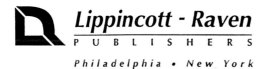

Lippincott - Raven
PUBLISHERS

Philadelphia • New York

Acquisitions Editor: Richard Winters
Sponsoring Editor: Melissa James
Associate Managing Editor: Grace R. Caputo
Production Manager: Caren Erlichman
Production Coordinator: David Yurkovich
Design Coordinator: Kathy Kelley-Luedtke
Interior Designer: Holly Reid McLaughlin
Cover Designer: Larry Pezzato
Indexer: Lynn E. Mahan
Compositor: Bi-Comp, Inc.
Printer/Binder: Walsworth Publishing Company

Printed in the United States of America

6 5 4 3

Library of Congress Cataloging-in-Publication Data

Rubin, Mark G.
    Manual of chemical peels: superficial and medium depth/by
Mark G. Rubin.
        p.   cm.
    Includes bibliographical references and index.
    ISBN 0-397-51506-5 (alk. paper)
    1. Chemical peel.
    [DNLM: 1. Chemexfoliation—methods. 2. Skin Aging. 3. Skin
Neoplasms—therapy.   QO 600 R896m 1995]
    RD520.R83 1995
    617.4'770592—dc20
    DNLM/DLC
    for Library of Congress   94-24385
                                                CIP

ACKNOWLEDGMENTS

Writing a book is an exciting yet arduous task. I want to thank my family—Jennifer, Lauren, and Mark, Jr.—as well as my office staff—Marcia, Kimberly, and Corey—for their support and understanding during this hectic and stressful time.

In addition, I thank Drs. Lee Kaplan and Charles Sexton for their helpful comments and criticisms. Thanks also go to Dr. James Dolezal for his contributions about each peeling agent.

Most importantly, I want to thank my father, Dr. Robert J. Rubin, for being the type of role model every physician should have. His high standards of ethics, concern for the patient's well-being, and desire to share his knowledge with others have been a major impetus in my writing this manual.

PREFACE

Superficial and medium depth skin peeling with trichloroacetic acid (TCA) has been a well-documented therapy in the United States since at least the 1960s. Some physicians were performing these peels earlier in this century, but the actual techniques and histology associated with them began to appear in the literature in the early 1960s with articles by Drs. Ayers and Resnick. TCA peels did not really become popular, however, until the late 1980s. Certainly, one of the reasons for this delay was that the population was not as interested in peels or as focused on antiaging processes before this time. Another reason is that in the early years of chemical peeling, most physicians did not prime the skin for several weeks before a peel and did not have the products for maintenance therapy that are now available. Therefore, their results were not as uniformly good as we are currently able to achieve. In addition, complications were more common and results were more transient.

Superficial and medium depth skin peels can create dramatic improvement in the skin, but their results are not as long lasting as those seen with phenol peels. The use of retinoic acid (Retin-A), alpha hydroxy acids, broad-spectrum sunscreens, and skin bleaches as part of a postpeel maintenance program has allowed patients to maintain the improvement in their skin for far longer. It is important not to approach superficial and medium depth skin peeling as a one-shot deal that fixes the patients' skin problems. Rather, these types of peels should be considered one step in an ongoing program of skin improvement. In reality, these peels are commonly repeated in order to achieve and maintain the best results.

I find it helpful to tell patients that the aging of skin is a chronic disease, like hypertension or diabetes. Just as these diseases need daily treatment to control or reverse them, so does aging skin. A single medium depth peel can reverse some of the clinical and histologic signs of aging, but once the skin has healed from the peel, the process of aging starts again. Therefore, a daily program of products designed to reverse the signs of aging is necessary to maintain long-term improvement.

There is no right or wrong way to treat photodamaged skin or to perform chemical peeling. A variety of peel techniques and agents are in use. I would encourage you to keep an open mind and to evaluate as many therapies as possible to find the least aggressive (and least risky) treatment regimens capable of producing the desired results.

The goal of *Manual of Chemical Peels* is not to make performing peels a totally "cookbook," step-by-step process, but rather to give you a rational scientific approach to using various chemicals to treat and improve photodamaged skin. It is not meant to be a heavily referenced textbook of peels. Instead, this manual attempts to lead you through the decision-making process in the chemical treatment of photodamaged skin. The section on basic concepts in skin peeling should provide you with a solid understanding of non-phenol peels. Feel free to copy or revise the patient information sheets and consent forms so that your office has all of the appropriate paperwork to handle patients undergoing peels. For best results, keep *Manual of Chemical Peels* in a readily available location in your office and refer to it frequently.

Mark G. Rubin, MD

CONTENTS

MANUAL OF CHEMICAL PEELS

Superficial and Medium Depth

Manual of Chemical Peels: Superficial and Medium Depth, by Mark G. Rubin.
J.B. Lippincott Company, Philadelphia, © 1995.

CHAPTER 1

PHOTOAGED AND PHOTODAMAGED SKIN

Classification of Skin Types and Levels of Photodamage ▶ *Assessment* ▶ *Dyschromias* ▶ *Wrinkles*

Aging is a dynamic process. As we age, certain histologic changes occur in our skin. These changes are induced by either intrinsic (chronologic) aging or extrinsic (environmental) aging.

Intrinsic aging changes are an inevitable part of the natural aging process of everyone's skin. The severity of some elements of chronologic aging may have a genetic basis, allowing some people's skin to age better than others. However, the most dramatic changes seen in aging skin are due to extrinsic causes.

By far the most significant environmental factor responsible for extrinsic aging is sunlight. The term *photoaging* denotes the aging changes due to chronic ultraviolet (UV) light exposure. The cumulative damage created by chronic UV light exposure, termed *photodamage*, can easily be seen by comparing the sun-exposed skin on the anterior chest with the sun-protected skin on the breast (Fig. 1-1).

It is well beyond the scope of this manual to address the numerous histologic and clinical changes associated with intrinsic and extrinsic aging. A brief summary of changes associated with photodamage is found below. The most significant clinical changes in photoaged skin versus sun protected skin are

- ▶ markedly increased roughness
- ▶ increased mottled hyperpigmentation
- ▶ increased loss of elasticity
- ▶ increased wrinkling

1

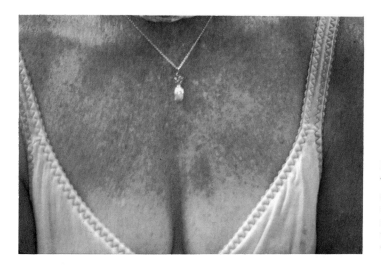

Figure 1-1
The skin on this patient is an excellent example of the difference between the sun-exposed anterior chest and the sun-protected skin on the breast.

Histologically, the changes seen in photodamaged skin are

▶ a thickened, more basket-woven stratum corneum
▶ a thinner, more atrophic epidermis
▶ epidermal atypia
▶ irregular dispersion of melanin throughout the epidermis
▶ decreased glycosaminoglycans in the dermis
▶ abnormal-appearing elastic fibers in the dermis

The goal of treating photodamage is to reverse these changes in the skin. Therefore, our goal is to create

▶ a thinner, more compact stratum corneum
▶ a thicker, acanthotic epidermis with no atypia and with a uniform dispersion of melanin
▶ increased deposition of new collagen and glycosaminoglycans in the dermis

▷ Classification of Skin Types and Levels of Photodamage

The most widely used classification of skin types in regard to chemical peeling has been the Fitzpatrick classification. It examines the ability of a patient's skin to tan or burn from UV light exposure. This information is helpful in determining which patients will respond well to chemical peeling and which have a high risk of pigmentation abnormalities from peels.

FITZPATRICK CLASSIFICATION SYSTEM

Skin Type	Skin Color	Characteristics
I	White	Always burns, never tans
II	White	Usually burns, tans less than average
III	White	Sometimes mild burn, tans about average
IV	White	Rarely burns, tans more than average
V	Brown	Rarely burns, tans profusely
VI	Black	Never burns, deeply pigmented

Patients can be classified as a certain Fitzpatrick skin type easily by asking them what happens when they are exposed to the sun. As a general rule, skin types I to III almost never develop postinflammatory hyperpigmentation, so these patients are excellent candidates for chemical peeling. Skin types IV to VI have significantly greater chance of developing postinflammatory hyperpigmentation. This does not mean that patients with these skin types cannot undergo peeling; they are just at a higher level of risk for pigmentation abnormalities.

Because superficial and medium depth nonphenol peels rarely create permanent hypopigmentation, patients of any skin type are able to have them, whereas those with skin types V and VI are often at risk for irregular hypopigmentation with deeper, phenol-based peels.

The Fitzpatrick classification is helpful for determining levels of risk of dyschromias associated with peels. However, it does not help us describe patients' type or level of photodamage. This information is helpful when trying to determine what needs to be corrected in a certain patient's skin. By allowing us to objectively compare the efficacy of different treatments, it is also helpful as a way to help standardize the science of chemical peeling and patient selection.

Several years ago, Dr. Richard Glogau introduced a classification system for photoaged skin. The concept of this system is to be able to objectively quantify the level of photodamage of the skin. This system has been helpful both in allowing physicians to standardize the approach to treating photodamaged skin and in aiding physicians to effectively communicate with one another about a given patient's level of damage.

GLOGAU CLASSIFICATION

Damage	Description	Characteristics
Type 1 (mild)	"No wrinkles"	Early photoaging • mild pigmentary changes • no keratoses • minimal wrinkles Patient age—20s or 30s • minimal or no makeup • minimal acne scarring
Type II (moderate)	"Wrinkles in motion"	Early to moderate photoaging • early senile lentigines visible • keratoses palpable but not visible • parallel smile lines beginning to appear Patient age—late 30s or 40s • some foundation usually worn • mild acne scarring
Type III (advanced)	"Wrinkles at rest"	Advanced photoaging • obvious dyschromia, telangiectasias • visible keratoses • wrinkles present even when not moving Patient age—50s or older • heavier foundation always worn • acne scarring present that makeup does not cover
Type IV (severe)	"Only wrinkles"	Severe photoaging • yellow—gray skin color • prior skin malignancies • wrinkles throughout, no normal skin Patient age—60s or 70s • makeup cannot be worn—it cakes and cracks • severe acne scarring

Although the Glogau system has been helpful in allowing us a more objective way to compare the efficacy of different treatments for certain skin types, I find it difficult to use for numerous reasons:

1. It tries to integrate acne scarring, wrinkling, and actinic keratoses—three distinctly different conditions.
2. It classifies patients according to the use of makeup, which varies widely among patients.
3. It fails to allow me to know how deep a peel is needed to correct the problem.

For example, if a 45-year-old woman with multiple visible actinic keratoses has almost no wrinkling, is she in group II or III?

I prefer to use a system that classifies the level of photodamage based on the histologic depth of visible clinical changes. This system allows the physician to identify the depth of the problems to be treated. Once the depth of the problem has been determined, it is easier to choose the type of depth-specific treatment. In other words, the classification system should make the selection of the appropriate therapy easier.

In addition, classifying photodamage in levels according to depth (or the depth of the peel necessary to correct it) allows you to easily predict the morbidity associated with the treatment program, which in turn facilitates patient discussions about the level of risk associated with the procedure. For example, a superficial intraepidermal peel is relatively risk free, whereas a reticular dermal peel has a significantly higher complication rate.

Based on this concept, I prefer to use a classification system that divides photodamage into three levels, as follows.

CLASSIFICATION OF PHOTODAMAGE

Level 1

Clinical signs are due to alteration in the epidermis only. Most abnormalities are of pigmentation and texture, including freckles, lentigines, and a dull, rough skin texture due to the increased thickness of the stratum corneum.

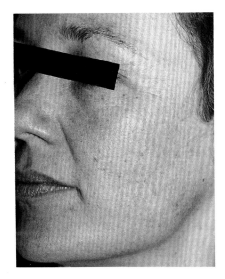

(continued)

CLASSIFICATION OF PHOTODAMAGE (Continued)

Level 2

Clinical signs are due to alterations of the epidermis and papillary dermis, and are also often related to abnormal pigmentation. Patients with level 2 damage may have all of the same clinical signs as those with level 1 damage. However, the textural and pigmentary changes are more marked. In addition, these patients may have actinic keratoses, liver spots (senile lentigines or flat seborrheic keratoses), and a definite increase in wrinkling. This increased wrinkling is usually seen in the infraorbital area and lateral to the nasolabial groove, where the skin may appear atrophic and crinkled.

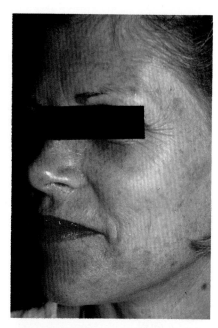

Level 3

Clinical signs are due to alterations in the epidermis, papillary dermis, and reticular dermis. The most severe form of photodamage, level 3 is associated with many of the clinical changes in level 1 and 2 changes. However, these patients also have marked wrinkling, usually associated with a thickened leathery appearance and feel, and often a yellowish tint to the skin. In addition, the skin of some patients has a pebbly texture and scattered open comedones.

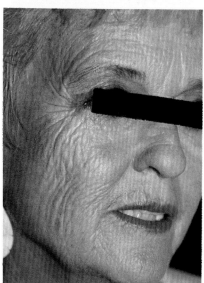

Obviously, as with all attempts at creating a classification system, this one is not perfect. Some patients may have problems in all three levels, others in only one or two. The important concept, however, is that a peel must be as deep as the deepest skin problem to achieve the best results. In other words, if the patient has some dyschromia located in the epidermis (level 1) and fine wrinkling due to papillary dermal atrophy and damage (level 2), he or she needs a peel that corrects papillary dermal damage to achieve the best results; an epidermal peel will improve the dyschromia but will have little or no impact on the wrinkling.

▷ Assessment

As stated earlier, the easiest approach to choosing the appropriate chemical peeling agent (and choosing the correct depth of peel) is to first determine the depth of peel needed. It is difficult, if not impossible, to determine the depth of hyperpigmentation using only clinical judgment and the naked eye. Therefore, it is helpful to have a Wood's lamp, or black light, which emits light at a wavelength of 354 nm (Fig. 1-2). Viewed under black light, areas of epidermal hyperpigmentation become more pronounced or accentuated, whereas areas of deeper dermal hyperpigmentation become less obvious. In simple terms, the worse a patient looks under a Wood's lamp, the more superficial the pigmentation and the easier it is to correct.

When using a Wood's lamp to evaluate hyperpigmentation, several points should be kept in mind to get the best results:

1. Always view the patient in as dark a room as possible. Even a small amount of ambient light makes it significantly more difficult to interpret the pigmentation abnormality and the results of the examination.
2. The angle of the lamp effects the accentuation of the pigmentation. I find it helpful to hold the lamp 8 to 12 inches from the patient's face

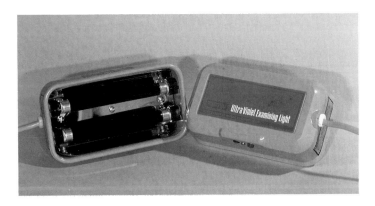

Figure 1-2
An example of a Wood's lamp.

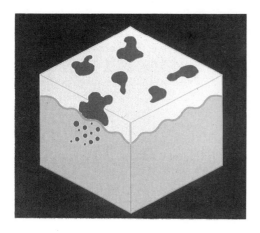

Figure 1-3

Diagram illustrating hyperpigmentation in the epidermis and dermis.

and to rotate my wrist at different angles while examining the area of hyperpigmentation. Changing the angle of the Wood's lamp like this can make the epidermal accentuation even more apparent.

3. Areas of hyperpigmentation that are accentuated by the Wood's lamp have epidermal melanin in them. In some cases, however, this melanin extends down into the dermis as well (Fig. 1-3). This is not apparent in the clinical view because of the intensified epidermal response to the Wood's lamp. This means that, because the superficial pigmentation may be obscuring a deeper melanin component, you can never be certain that removal of the epidermis will completely remove an area of hyperpigmentation accentuated by a Wood's lamp.

4. The intensity of the Wood's lamp directly affects the degree of pigmentation accentuation. The battery-powered lamps and lamps with only one bulb are definitely not as effective as the lamps with two bulbs that plug into a wall outlet.

▷ Dyschromias

The two most common complaints bringing patients into a doctor's office for a peel consultation are wrinkles and dyschromias. Both of these conditions are commonly associated with excessive sun exposure and photodamage.

Dyschromias are alterations in pigmentation, most commonly hyperpigmentation. Various hyperpigmented lesions are commonly seen on the skin of patients with photodamage. It is important to closely examine each lesion and to determine its depth in the skin. Once you know how deep it is, you know how deep a peel is needed to remove it.

The hyperpigmented lesions most commonly seen are ephelides (freckles), lentigines simplex, senile lentigines, flat seborrheic keratoses, nevi, melasma, and postinflammatory hyperpigmentation. Let's approach these one at a time and examine what these lesions look like both clinically and histologically.

Freckles (Ephelides)

Clinical Findings
▶ Small brown macules on sun-exposed areas, which darken with sun exposure

Histology
▶ Normal epidermal architecture without elongation of rete ridges
▶ Increased melanin along the basal cell layer
▶ Melanocytes normal in number but larger and more dendritic

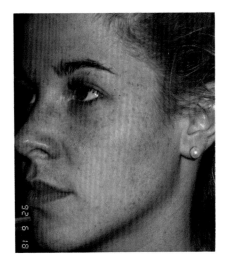

Lentigines Simplex

Clinical Findings
▶ Small, evenly pigmented, light to dark brown macules on sun-exposed or non–sun-exposed areas; similar in appearance to junctional nevi

Histology
▶ Slight elongation of rete ridges
▶ Increase in melanocytes and melanin in basal regional or above
▶ Melanophages in the upper dermis

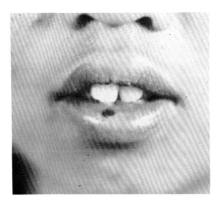

Senile (Solar) Lentigines

Clinical Findings

▶ Dark brown macules of various sizes on sun-exposed areas of older individuals; usually with irregular borders

Histology

▶ Clublike elongation of rete ridges with possible areas of atrophic epidermis
▶ More numerous melanocytes with increased melanin
▶ Melanophages in upper dermis

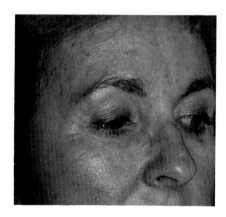

Seborrheic Keratoses

Clinical Findings

▶ Slightly raised to thickened, light brown to black lesions in various sites; often appear to be "stuck on"

Histology

▶ Marked increase in thickness of squamous and stratum corneum layers
▶ Varied amounts of pigmentation, primarily in basal layer but often throughout the epidermis

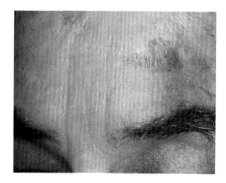

Junctional Nevi

Clinical Findings
▶ Well-demarcated, light to dark brown macules occurring anywhere on the body

Histology
▶ Numerous single and clustered nevus cells (nondendritic melanocytes) along the dermal–epidermal junction or bulging into the dermis
▶ Varied amount of pigment seen in the nevus cells, epidermis, and dermal melanophages

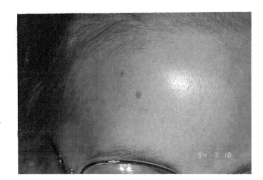

Melasma

Clinical Findings
▶ Symmetric, sharply demarcated, irregular patches of light to dark hyperpigmentation; usually seen on the face

Histology
▶ Increased melanocytes and melanin in the basal and suprabasal layers
▶ Dermal melanophages present in various degrees

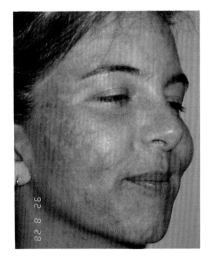

Postinflammatory Hyperpigmentation

Clinical Findings
▶ Poorly demarcated hyper-pigmented macules in areas of previous inflammation

Histology
▶ Increased melanin in the epidermis with or without dermal melanophages

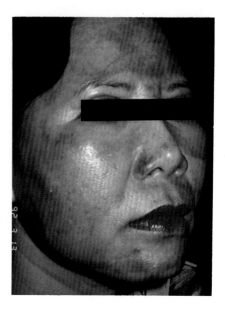

A review of the histology of these lesions should make it clear why certain lesions respond better to light peels than others and why some lesions do not respond well to even a medium depth peel.

To achieve the best results for your patients, there are several points to keep in mind:

1. When treating melasma or postinflammatory hyperpigmentation, always examine the skin with a Wood's lamp to determine whether the pigmentation is epidermal or dermal. This is of utmost importance, since dermal pigmentation will not respond to epidermal peeling.

2. If you attempt to treat postinflammatory hyperpigmentation with peeling, be careful not to induce too much inflammation with the peel or you may stimulate more hyperpigmentation.

3. Do not attempt to improve hyperpigmented nevi with light or medium depth peels, to which they generally do not respond well. Nevus cells are resistant to peeling agents and occasionally even darken after a peel.

4. Liver spots or age spots can be forms of senile lentigines or seborrheic keratoses. Both of these lesions are epidermal, but they extend finger-like projections down into the upper dermis. Therefore, an epidermal peel will leave behind the tips of these projections, and these lesions will recur.

5. Palpable seborrheic keratoses have so much hyperkeratosis and thickening of the epidermis that most acids (other than alpha hydroxy acids) do not penetrate well into these lesions. Other treatment modalities, such as cryotherapy, are needed before or after a peel to give the best results.

Summary of Peel Results

Epidermal Peels

Excellent Results
▶ Ephelides
▶ Epidermal melasma
▶ Epidermal hyperpigmentation

Variable Results
▶ Lentigines simplex
▶ Senile lentigines
▶ Mixed (epidermal and dermal) melasma
▶ Mixed postinflammatory hyperpigmentation

Poor Results
▶ Seborrheic keratoses
▶ Junctional nevi
▶ Dermal melasma
▶ Dermal postinflammatory hyperpigmentation

Papillary Dermal Peels

Excellent Results
▶ Ephelides
▶ Lentigines simplex
▶ Senile lentigines
▶ Epidermal melasma
▶ Epidermal postinflammatory hyperpigmentation

Variable Results
▶ Seborrheic keratoses
▶ Dermal and mixed melasma
▶ Dermal and mixed postinflammatory hyperpigmentation

Poor Results
▶ Nevi
▶ Some exophytic seborrheic keratoses

The reason that seborrheic keratoses, which are epidermal lesions, may not respond to papillary dermal peeling is that the acid may not penetrate through the keratoses and may create only an intraepidermal peel in that area. The reason for variable results with mixed or dermal melasma and postinflammatory hyperpigmentation is that melanophages in these conditions may extend beyond the papillary dermis.

Although postinflammatory hyperpigmentation and melasma are two separate entities, their treatment is often similar. As with the treatment of all other hyperpigmented lesions, there are two key points:

1. Block the creation of more melanin, which continually "feeds" the dark lesion.
2. Exfoliate the epidermis to decrease the number of melanin granules present.

A detailed discussion of the treatment of melasma and postinflammatory hyperpigmentation can be found in Chapters 10 and 11 (section on patient selection).

▷ Wrinkles

Few lesions are as universally feared and disliked as wrinkles. Unfortunately, the exact mechanism of formation of wrinkles is not completely understood. However, there are several theories:

Fine wrinkles or crinkles—presumably due to thinning of the epidermis and upper dermis, creating a "cigarette paper" type of tissue that crinkles easily. These lines often appear as crosshatched wrinkling (Fig. 1-4).

Muscle-related wrinkles—caused by repetitive movements that create a "dent" in the epidermis and most of the dermis. These are akin to the creases or dents that can be created by repeatedly folding a sheet of metal back and forth (see Fig. 1-4).

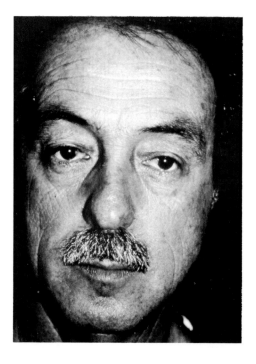

Figure 1-4
Muscle-related lines on the forehead are contrasted with fine lines (seen as crosshatched wrinkles) in the infraorbital and malar area.

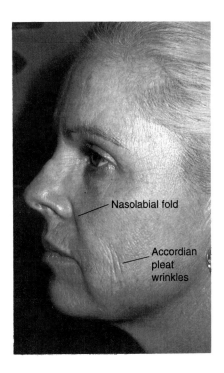

Nasolabial fold

Accordian pleat wrinkles

Figure 1-5
Accordion pleat wrinkles (parallel smile lines) on the cheek of a patient with severe actinic damage. In addition, a fold can be seen in the nasolabial area.

> *Accordion pleat wrinkles*—due to loose redundant skin with atrophy of the epidermis, dermis, and subcutaneous tissue, as well as loss of elasticity (Fig. 1-5)
> *Folds*—due to the downward sagging of the skin and underlying muscles that is caused by gravity (see Fig. 1-5)

The idea here again is to closely examine the skin, determine the type of problem (wrinkles), and decide what it is due to and then formulate the best plan for correcting it.

Peels have the ability to create a thicker epidermis, more collagen in the papillary and reticular dermis, more glycosaminoglycans in the papillary and reticular dermis, and more elastic staining fibers in the dermis. The end result of these histologic changes is an increased volume of tissue, which tightens the superficial skin layers, leading to improvement of the wrinkles. The dermal changes are directly proportional to the depth of the peel; that is, the deeper the peel, the more collagen and glycosaminoglycan deposition. Therefore, lighter peels can help the more superficial types of wrinkles, but a deeper type of peel, with its resultant significant increases in new collagen and glycosaminoglycans, is usually necessary to improve deep lines.

Some evidence suggests that repetitive superficial intraepidermal peels can create new collagen deposition in the dermis. This explains why repeated light peels can help some wrinkles. However, it is incorrect to extrapolate this information and state that multiple light peels can equal the effect of one deeper peel. It is important to realize that **repeated light or even medium depth peels do not create any change in the reticular dermis that comes close to approximating the change induced by a deep peel.** Thus, lighter peels do not improve deep lines the way a reticular dermal peel does. I have seen patients with muscle-related wrinkles that are essentially unchanged after six yearly papillary dermal trichloroacetic acid (TCA) peels.

It has been my experience that only wrinkles due to atrophy respond well to nonphenol (superficial and medium depth) peeling. Wrinkles due to gravitational effects or muscle movement require reticular dermal peels or other therapies to be appropriately treated. It is usually a waste of your time and the patient's to treat deep wrinkles with lighter peels.

Once you have identified the level of photodamage, you are in a position to choose an appropriate treatment regimen. Often, several treatment options can achieve the desired results. Later chapters in this manual explore the available therapeutic options, including both the various levels of skin peels and several nonpeeling therapies for the treatment of photodamage.

Manual of Chemical Peels: Superficial and Medium Depth, by Mark G. Rubin.
J.B. Lippincott Company, Philadelphia, © 1995.

CHAPTER 2

WHAT ARE SKIN PEELS?

Classifications of Peel Depths ▶ *Peeling Agents* ▶ *Toxicity*

Skin is a dynamic, growing organ. Every day cells divide at the basal layer of the epidermis and begin their journey upward to the uppermost layer, the stratum corneum. As new cells continue to grow, old cells from the stratum corneum slough off (Fig. 2-1). This exfoliation of cells from the stratum corneum is a normal daily event.

Chemical peeling is basically an accelerated form of exfoliation induced by the use of a chemical cauterant or escharotic agent. Very light peeling agents induce a faster sloughing of the cells in the stratum corneum, whereas deeper peeling agents create necrosis and inflammation in the epidermis, papillary dermis, or reticular dermis (Fig. 2-2).

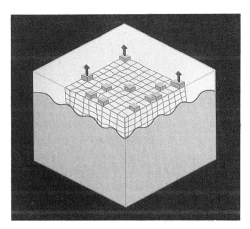

Figure 2-1

Haphazard shedding of cells from the stratum corneum.

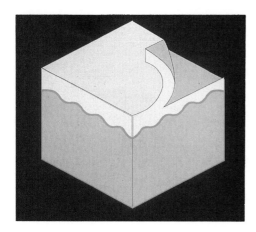

Figure 2-2
Uniform level of necrosis and peeling induced by a
chemical peel.

Chemical peeling creates changes in skin through three mechanisms:

▶ Stimulation of epidermal growth through removal of the stratum corneum. Even very light peels that do not create necrosis of "the living
epidermis" can induce the epidermis to thicken.

▶ Destruction of specific layers of damaged skin. By destroying the layers
and replacing them with more "normalized" tissue, a better cosmetic
result is achieved. This is especially true in the treatment of pigmentation abnormalities and actinic keratoses.

▶ Induction of an inflammatory reaction deeper in the tissue than the
necrosis induced by the peeling agent. Activation of the mediators of
inflammation (through a poorly understood mechanism) is able to induce production of new collagen and ground substance in the dermis.
Epidermal wounds are capable of inducing deposition of collagen and
glycosaminoglycans in the dermis.

Because deeper peels involve a greater risk of complication and a longer period of
recovery, or downtime, the goal is to create as little necrosis as possible while
inducing as much new tissue formation as possible. This is the concept behind
repetitive superficial and medium depth peels. They have low risk, but they create
cumulative benefits that far exceed the results of one lighter peel.

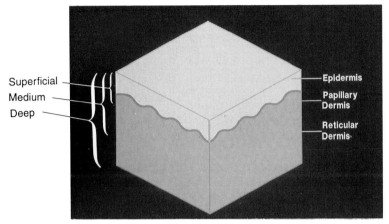

Figure 2-3
Old classification of peel depths: superficial peel destruction from the epidermis to the papillary dermis, medium depth peels destruction to the upper reticular dermis, deep peels destruction to the mid-reticular dermis.

▷ Classification of Peel Depths

Most recent articles on chemical peeling offer the same classification of depth of peels (Fig. 2-3):

> *Superficial peels*—destruction anywhere from the epidermis to the papillary dermis
> *Medium depth peels*—destruction extending to the upper reticular dermis
> *Deep peels*—destruction extending to the mid-reticular dermis

I don't think this classification is an effective one. Peels of the epidermis, papillary dermis, or reticular dermis differ significantly in their benefits and risks. A "superficial peel" to the level of the stratum corneum is an extremely different peel from a "superficial peel" to the level of the papillary dermis.

Therefore, in keeping with my preferred classification of photodamaged skin (outlined in Chapter 1), I offer here a simple but effective classification of peel depths. To begin, divide the levels of peels into four groups, based on the histologic boundaries of the level of necrosis. This allows you to easily predict the following:

> *What will improve from that level of peel?* If you know from your photodamage classification how deep the patient's skin abnormalities are, you also know how deep a peel is needed to correct them. For example, if the patient has epidermal hyperpigmentation, a stratum corneum peel

would not be sufficient to correct it, but a full-thickness epidermal peel would be. Similarly, if the patient has papillary dermal elastosis and atrophy with wrinkling, an epidermal peel is insufficient to correct this.

What effect will this peel have on the patient's life-style? The deeper the peel, the more unsightly the patient's appearance soon afterward. A stratum corneum peel allows patients to function normally in their daily lives, whereas a papillary dermal peel—with its associated erythema, edema, and hyperpigmentation—prevents most patients from performing their normal social or job-related functions for a full week.

What risks are associated with this peel? Basically, the deeper the peel, the greater the risk of complications. If you never peel below the epidermis, it is essentially impossible to create scarring or hypopigmentation (unless an infection develops). Similarly, any peel into the reticular dermis results in some degree of hypopigmentation.

$\triangledown$

LEVELS OF PEELS (FIG. 2-4)

Very superficial (exfoliation): These peels thin or remove the stratum corneum and do not create a wound below the stratum granulosum.
Superficial (epidermal): These peels create necrosis of part or all of the epidermis, anywhere from the stratum granulosum to the basal cell layer.
Medium (papillary dermal): These peels create necrosis of the epidermis and part or all of the papillary dermis.
Deep (reticular dermal): These peels create necrosis of the epidermis and papillary dermis, which extends into the reticular dermis.

$\triangle$

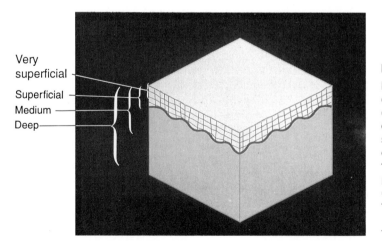

Very
superficial
Superficial
Medium
Deep

Figure 2-4

New classification of peel depths: *very superficial*—destruction of the stratum corneum; *superficial*—destruction of part or all of the epidermis; *medium*—destruction of the epidermis and part or all of the papillary dermis; *deep*—destruction of the epidermis and the papillary dermis that extends into the reticular dermis.

▷ Peeling Agents

- ▶ Retinoic acid (Retin A)
- ▶ 5-Fluorouracil (5-FU)
- ▶ Jessner's solution
- ▶ Resorcinol
- ▶ Salicylic acid
- ▶ Trichloroacetic acid (TCA)
- ▶ Alpha hydroxy acids (AHAs)
- ▶ Alpha keto acids (pyruvic acid)
- ▶ Phenol

When the term *peeling agent* is used in this book, I am really referring to an agent that can induce some form of peeling after one application. Therefore, although retinoic acid and 5-FU can create very superficial peels after repeated use, they really should not be referred to as true peeling agents.

It is difficult to definitively classify the remaining peeling agents as very superficial, superficial, medium, or deep peeling agents. The depth of a peel depends on many variables, including

- ▶ the peeling agent
- ▶ the concentration of the peeling agent
- ▶ how many coats of the agent are applied
- ▶ the technique of application (ie, painted on or rubbed in)
- ▶ how the skin was cleaned and degreased before the peel
- ▶ how the skin was primed in the weeks preceding the peel
- ▶ the type of skin the patient has (ie, thin, thick)
- ▶ the anatomic location of the peel
- ▶ the duration of contact with the skin (particularly AHAs)

With so many variables related to the depth of the peel, any classification of peeling agents can be only approximate, since an agent that produces a superficial peel in one patient may produce a medium depth peel in another.

As an example, application of 25% TCA with a cotton-tipped swab to the face of a man with oily, thick skin that was not primed before the peel will create a superficial intraepidermal peel. On the other hand, if a gauze square saturated with 25% TCA is repeatedly rubbed on the face of a thin-skinned woman who has been applying 0.1% retinoic acid cream twice daily for 2 weeks, the peel that results will be much deeper, probably medium depth, extending into the papillary dermis. Therefore, you could correctly state that 25% TCA can be a superficial or medium depth peeling agent.

For the sake of simplicity, you should always try to standardize your peel, no matter what peeling agent you use: prime all patients in a similar manner, clean their skin in a similar manner, and apply the acid in a similar manner. By standardizing your technique, you will decrease the number of variables that can inadvertently change the depth of the peel. Assuming that patients are primed and cleaned (degreased) in a similar manner, the following classification system is fairly reliable.

CLASSIFICATION OF PEELING AGENTS

Very Superficial

Glycolic acid 30% to 50% applied briefly (1 to 2 minutes)
Jessner's solution applied in 1 to 3 coats
Low-concentration resorcinol 20% to 30% applied briefly (5 to 10 minutes)
TCA 10% applied in 1 coat

Superficial

Glycolic acid 50% to 70% applied for a variable time (2 to 20 minutes)
Jessner's solution applied in 4 to 10 coats
Resorcinol 40% to 50% applied for 30 to 60 minutes
TCA 10% to 30%

Medium Depth

Glycolic acid 70% applied for a variable time (3 to 30 minutes)
TCA 35% to 50%
Augmented TCA (CO_2 plus TCA 35%; Jessner's solution plus TCA 35%; glycolic acid 70% plus TCA 35%)

Deep

Phenol 88%
Baker Gordon Phenol Formula

▷ Toxicity

As a general rule, nonphenol peels carry a significantly lesser risk of toxicity than phenol peels.

At this time, there are no reported cases of systemic toxicity from TCA or AHAs. This does not mean that these chemicals are necessarily free from systemic reaction. I have seen one case of urticaria associated with a 35% TCA peel. This was later shown to be cholinergic urticaria triggered by the tachycardia and flushing associated with the TCA peel. In addition, some patients may feel faint or light-headed during their peel because of the accompanying facial vasodilation and tachycardia. It is common to see marked mottled hyperemia on the neck and chest of a patient undergoing medium depth TCA peeling (Fig. 2-5).

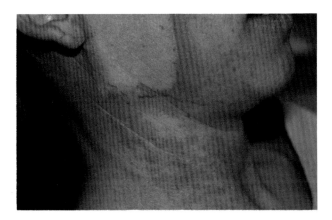

Figure 2-5

Mottled reactive hyperemia on the neck of a patient undergoing a 30% TCA facial peel.

I have seen two cases of allergic reactions to lactic acid peels performed by nonphysicians. In neither case was I able to get the list of all the ingredients in the peeling agent. Therefore, it is possible that the reactions were due to another chemical in the peeling solution rather than to the lactic acid itself. This is probable, in fact, since I have never seen an allergic reaction to low-dose lactic acid creams (or to Jessner's solution, which contains 14% lactic acid), which I have been using for more than a decade.

Two nonphenol chemical peeling agents have the potential for systemic toxicity—resorcinol and salicylic acid. In the literature, it has been repeatedly stated that the surface area peeled with Jessner's solution must be limited because of the potential toxicity of resorcinol (Jessner's solution is 14 g resorcinol, 14 g salicylic acid, and 14 g lactic acid [USP 85%] in ethanol to make 100 mL). It has been suggested that, to prevent this toxicity, Jessner's solution not be used over large surface areas, such as the chest or back, at the same time as it is used on the face. The contradiction here is that 40% or 50% resorcinol peels are routinely performed on the back or chest without toxicity, and these have three times the concentration of resorcinol as Jessner's solution.

In reality, the limiting factor in using Jessner's peels over large areas appears to be the degree of absorption of salicylic acid with resultant salicylism. Salicylism is not that uncommon if multiple areas are peeled at one time (ie, the face, neck, chest, and arms).

Since this book is a practical manual, let's look at "real-life" toxicity problems due to these chemicals and consider how to deal with them.

Resorcinol Toxicity

Resorcinol has been shown to cause death in rare instances when used as follows: 40% paste applied daily for 1 to 4 hours for 22 to 23 days, which also causes tremors, collapse, and violet-black urine. Resorcinol has also been reported to cause methemoglobinemia, methemoglubinuria, hypothyroidism, syncope, and circulatory collapse. In addition, it has been repeatedly stated that a high percentage of the population is allergic to resorcinol. This is a particularly interesting comment in view of the fact that I have performed more than 1000 peels with Jessner's solution and have never seen a case of allergic contact dermatitis resulting from it.

Resorcinol peeling is popular in many other countries. Despite the large number of such peels being performed, only a handful of patients have experienced serious toxicity. You should be aware of the potential toxicity, but the odds of your having to deal with a toxic reaction are extremely small. If carefully observed, the following two guidelines should help you avoid any serious problems from the use of resorcinol:

Rule #1   Always do a small patch test application of any peeling solution or paste containing resorcinol several days before the actual peel. This will help you detect anyone with a sensitivity to resorcinol.

Apply the compound in the postauricular area for 15 minutes and examine the spot 2 days later. Any evidence of vesiculation or marked edema implies possible contact sensitivity; such patients should not undergo resorcinol peeling. Mild erythema may be present as a normal response to resorcinol.

Rule #2   Because peeling compounds containing resorcinol have a tendency to produce marked vasodilation, patients undergoing resorcinol peels may become light-headed or even syncopal. Always perform resorcinol peeling with the patients lying down, and have them get up slowly after the peel.

Salicylism

Salicylic acid is another phenol derivative. Its toxicity is referred to as *salicylism*. Absorption of enough salicylic acid can cause death, as has been reported with 20% salicylic acid in an alcohol solution applied twice in 1 day to 50% of the body. Lesser levels of toxicity are more common, including rapid breathing, tinnitus, decreased hearing, and dizziness. Nausea, vomiting, and abdominal cramps may also occur. More severe toxic reactions are marked by more serious central nervous system reactions, with mental disturbances that can simulate alcohol intoxication. Allergic reactions to salicylic acid are extremely rare, so patch testing is not required before peeling.

Salicylic acid is safe as a peeling agent, as long as you exercise caution. Follow these guidelines and you shouldn't have any problems:

1. Do not peel large areas with salicylic acid solutions or pastes.
   a. Because Jessner's solution contains 14% salicylic acid, applying it to the face, neck, chest, and arms means that over 25% of the body has been peeled and there is a good chance of salicylism.
   b. A 40% salicylic acid paste has about three times the concentration of salicylic acid as Jessner's solution, and it is used under occlusion, which enhances its penetration. Therefore, peel only small areas when using salicylic acid paste (eg, peel only one arm at a time).
2. In patients with kidney disease, who are unable to excrete salicylic acid as rapidly as healthier patients, the risk of toxicity is increased. In these patients, avoid salicylic acid, or peel only very small areas at a time (eg, a dorsal hand, followed later by the dorsal forearm).
3. Have all patients undergoing peels containing salicylic acid drink at least eight glasses of water during the first 12 hours after the peel. This will help with the excretion of the salicylic acid.
4. Warn patients to notify you as soon as possible if they experience any light-headedness or tinnitus after salicylic acid peels. If so, instruct them to remove any salicylic acid paste still on their skin and to increase their intake of oral fluids; in more severe cases, consider meeting them in the emergency department, where intravenous fluids can be rapidly administered and urine alkalinization performed.

Manual of Chemical Peels: Superficial and Medium Depth, by Mark G. Rubin. J.B. Lippincott Company, Philadelphia, © 1995.

CHAPTER **3**

REVERSAL OF PHOTODAMAGE WITH CHEMICAL NONPEEL TECHNIQUES

Sun Avoidance ▸ *Retinoic Acid* ▸ *Alpha Hydroxy Acids* ▸ *Combination Therapy* ▸ *Other Nonpeel Methods*

Although a peel may be an excellent therapy for a patient, not all patients are interested in undergoing peels. Some are afraid of the whole concept of peeling, or they may have had a bad experience with a previous peel. Other patients may not have the time to heal from a peel.

Fortunately, there are some nonpeel treatments available to improve photo-damaged skin. These products are commonly used in conjunction with chemical peeling as part of the maintenance program of skin care after a peel. In some patients, however, the use of these products alone, without chemical peeling, can provide acceptable results.

▷ Sun Avoidance

The first step in any program of treating photodamaged skin is to stop on-going photodamage. It makes little sense to improve the quality of the skin and then subject it to further damage from chronic ultraviolet (UV) light exposure.

Early studies by Kligman showed that complete avoidance of sunlight for several years can actually reverse some histologic signs of photodamage. In other words, the skin has the ability to repair itself if it is protected from continual photodamage.

In reality, total sun avoidance is difficult if not impossible for most people. Therefore, we must settle for the next best thing—sun protection. The concept of sun protection encompasses sun protective clothing (including hats) and sunscreens.

The easiest to use and most reasonable protection for most people is sunscreen. Sunscreen should be worn every day, whether the person is outdoors a little or a lot. Because UV damage is cumulative in its effects, the prevention of even small daily amounts of sun damage over a long period of time can have a profound impact on the total amount of UV-induced damage.

It is also important to consider the type of sunscreen being used. Basically, they can be broken down into two types—physical blocks and chemical blocks. *Physical blocks* actually create a physical barrier to the penetration of UV light into the skin. The classic physical block is zinc oxide or titanium dioxide, long popular with lifeguards to protect their noses and lips. More recently, these products benefitted from the addition of bright colors to the paste, thus allowing youngsters to paint their faces with a rainbow of colors.

Although physical blocks are effective, they are not cosmetically elegant. Most patients are unwilling to wear these products daily. Recently, some products containing micronized titanium dioxide have become available. When applied, these physical blocks do not appear as an opaque cream but rather as a filmy or slightly powdery layer, which most patients find much more acceptable than their old counterparts. The benefits of these products are that they provide very broad-spectrum coverage and are less irritating to sensitive skin types than traditional chemical sunscreens. Nevertheless, sunblocks containing micronized titanium dioxide are still not as cosmetically appealing as the chemical sunscreens and must be applied in a fairly thick layer to work their best. Examples of these products include Neutrogena Chemical-Free Sunblocker SPF 17 and Ti-Screen Natural SPF 16.

Chemical sunscreens rely on the absorption of UV light by the active "sunscreen chemical." Once the absorbing chemical binds to the stratum corneum, it prevents the penetration of UV light into the deeper layers of the skin. The most popular sunscreen had been para-aminobenzoic acid (PABA). It has since been replaced by other chemicals because of its tendency to create staining, its fairly high rate of contact allergy, and its inability to block any UVA light.

Newer sunscreens generally contain several active chemical agents in an effort to provide broad-spectrum protection. Most sunscreens are aimed at blocking UVB (280 to 320 nm) light, since these wavelengths are thought to be the most carcinogenic. The sun protection factor (SPF) number on a bottle of sunscreen is actually a measure of how effective the sunscreen is in being able to block erythema induced by UVB light. Research has shown that sunscreens with an SPF of 15 actually block about 92% to 94% of the UVB light. It is important to be aware that most patients apply only half the amount of sunscreen (1 mg/cm^2) used by researchers when testing an SPF (2 mg/cm^2). Therefore, you need to encourage your patients to apply their sunscreen more thickly than normal for the best protection.

Recently, there has been a stronger focus on protection from UVA (320 to 360 nm) light as well. On-going studies have suggested that these wavelengths of light are not as benign as they were initially believed to be. Therefore, newer sunscreens are often labeled "broad-spectrum coverage" implying that they block UVA as well as UVB light. Unfortunately, at this time there is no FDA-regulated rating system (equivalent to the SPF system) that demonstrates the level of a product's UVA-blocking ability. At this time, it appears that Parsol 1789 is the best UVA-blocking agent available in this country. Other chemicals, including anthranilates and benzophenones, seem to be effective as well, but not to the same degree as Parsol 1789.

FDA-Approved Sunscreen Agents

Ultraviolet A Absorbers

Oxybenzone
Sulisobenzone
Dioxybenzone
Menthyl anthranilate
Avobenzone
Butylmethoxydibenzoylmethane

Ultraviolet B Absorbers

Aminobenzoic acid
Amyl dimethyl PABA
2-Ethoxyethyl p-methoxycinnamate
Diethanolamine p-methoxycinnamate
Digalloyl trioleate
Ethyl 4-bis (hydroxypropyl) aminobenzoate
2-Ethylhexyl-2-cyano-3,3-diphenyl-acrylate
Ethylhexyl salicylate
Glyceryl aminobenzoate
Homomenthyl salicylate
Lawsone with dihydroxyacetone
Octyl dimethyl PABA
2-Phenylbenzimidazole-5-sulfonic acid
Triethanolamine salicylate

Blocking UVA and UVB light is important in treating photodamage. Because UVA light penetrates deeper into the skin than UVB light, it appears to play a significant role in actinically induced wrinkling and damage to the dermis. In addition, UVA light (often called "tanning rays") can readily intensify hyperpigmentation of the skin, including ephelides, melasma, and postinflammatory hyperpigmentation. This effect can be so dramatic that many patients with hyperpigmentation improve significantly when they change from daily use of a UVB-blocking sunscreen to daily use of a broad-spectrum sunscreen.

What this all means in basic terms is that **daily use of a broad-spectrum sunscreen is imperative in the treatment of photodamaged skin.** Significant amounts of UVA light pass through window glass, so patients who are indoors near a window all day are still getting UV exposure and should wear a broad-spectrum sunscreen. The exact type or brand of sunscreen is a matter of patient and physician preference. Some patients prefer a gel, others a cream, and so forth. However, for most of my patients, I recommend a moisturizer-based, broad-spectrum sunscreen containing Parsol 1789 (eg, Shade UVA Guard) each morning.

For patients who are subject to extreme amounts of sun exposure (eg, skiing, mountain climbing, sailing), I encourage the application of a broad-spectrum chemical sunscreen each morning, followed 20 to 30 minutes later by the application of a titanium dioxide, chemical-free sunscreen. This double layer of sunscreens gives patients the benefit of both a chemical and a physical screening agent.

Patients should be reminded to wear sunscreen daily on all exposed areas. It is particularly important to apply a broad-spectrum sunscreen to the neck, chest, and dorsal hands in addition to the face. Failure to block UVA exposure to these areas makes that skin appear darker and more aged than the skin of the face. This all too familiar look of a youthful face and a weathered chest, neck, and hands is the telltale sign of a previous cosmetic procedure having been performed on the face. This is the reason to consider treating the neck, hands, and often the chest with a skin care maintenance program similar to that for the face. All areas of visible sun damage should be treated to achieve the best cosmetic results.

▷ Retinoic Acid

Retinoic acid (tretinoin; Retin-A) has really triggered the revolution of the non-surgical treatment for sun-damaged skin. Before the introduction of "Retin-A for wrinkles," chemical peels were not particularly popular and there were really no scientifically proven topical therapies for photoaging. When the lay press began to hype retinoic acid for the treatment of aging skin, millions of people went to their doctors in an effort to improve the look of their skin. Once such behavior became socially acceptable rather than a symbol of extreme vanity, it opened the door to other therapies. Interest in light and medium depth peels exploded as retinoic acid users began to request faster and more significant improvements in their skin than they were achieving on regimens of retinoic acid alone.

Retinoic acid has withstood the test of time. Considerable scientific research shows that it improves the histologic signs of photoaging and photodamage. Most long-term retinoic acid users also demonstrate some degree of clinical improvement in their skin.

There are three problems with retinoic acid:

1. The ability of retinoic acid to correct wrinkles was overplayed in the lay press, and patients began to expect too much from the product. These disappointed patients started the avalanche of negative press about retinoic acid seen in the early 1990s.

2. Retinoic acid is not a user-friendly drug. Most patients who use it have an initial period of retinoid dermatitis that lasts several weeks. During this time, their skin is red, peeling, and sensitive. Once the dermatitis has subsided and the skin has acclimated to retinoic acid use, a significant number of patients still have occasional mild relapses of dermatitis, usually lasting only 1 or 2 days. This can occur even after several years of use.

   In addition, patients who use retinoic acid demonstrate a degree of increased photosensitivity. In some cases, this may be heat-triggered facial flushing rather than true photosensitivity. However, despite wearing a sunscreen, patients who are outdoors a great deal often complain of a burning sensation on their face while in the sun. They are often more comfortable if they wear a sunblock containing a physical blocking agent like titanium dioxide, as well as a hat.

3. Retinoic acid increases capillary arborization in the dermis. This increased blood flow to the face is often characterized as a healthy rosy glow. However, the same effect may worsen existing facial telangiectasia or may keep the patient's face red. Retinoic acid use should be avoided or minimized in patients with ruddy complexions, easy facial flushing, or facial telangiectasia.

Is there a place for retinoic acid in the chemical treatment of photodamaged skin? Absolutely! Research has shown that there are specific retinoid receptors in the skin, leading to the belief that some of the effects of retinoic acid are specific to that agent alone. However, now that we have access to other chemicals (including alpha hydroxy acids and superficial chemical peeling agents) retinoic acid does not have to be the mainstay of a treatment program.

WHAT DOES RETINOIC ACID ACTUALLY DO?

Histologically	Clinically
Thins and compacts the stratum corneum	Results in smoother, softer skin texture
Thickens the epidermis	Tightens the skin
Reverses keratinocyte atypia	Improves or eradicates actinic keratoses
Disperses melanin throughout epidermis	Improves blotchy hyperpigmentation
Stimulates dermal collagen deposition	Increases dermal volume and tightens the skin
Increases glycosaminoglycan deposition	Increases dermal volume and tightens the skin
Increases neovascularization in dermis	Gives a pinker, rosy hue to the skin

Using Retinoic Acid

Retinoic acid is available in the following forms; each tube has a colored stripe on the end corresponding to its strength:

> *Cream*—0.025% (gray), 0.05% (blue), 0.1% (red)
> *Gel*—0.01% (green), 0.025% (orange)
> *Liquid*—0.05%

The creams are in a moisturizing base, so this form of Retin-A is preferred for patients with mature, dry skin. The gels contain alcohol, and although the percentage of retinoic acid in them is lower than in the creams, the gel base enhances the penetration of the acid. In addition, the gel is drying by nature and often irritates adult skin. The liquid contains alcohol and is very drying, so it is rarely used on adult skin. On occasion, I use the liquid on patients with very thick sebaceous skin, but most people cannot tolerate it.

There are two approaches to using retinoic acid—conservative and aggressive. In patients with sensitive skin and mild photodamage, a conservative therapy usually works quite well. However, for patients with thick, tough skin or severe sun damage, a conservative approach is of little or no value.

It is better to prescribe daily use of retinoic acid than alternate-day therapy. My experience suggests that patients who use retinoic acid everyday acclimate faster and better to it. If a patient has been using retinoic acid routinely and then discontinues it for a week or so, it takes at least 1 to 2 weeks to get him or her reacclimated to the product. I think this same phenomenon exists to a lesser degree in patients who use it every second or third day: they have difficulty stabilizing on retinoic acid and seem to have more trouble, with some degree of chronic peeling. Therefore, **have patients try to use retinoic acid every night, even if it has to be diluted.** Because you do not know what strength retinoic acid the patient will ultimately use, it is wise to initially write a prescription for the smaller 20-g tube rather than the 45-g tube. The best idea is to give the patient a sample to try first.

Patients With Sensitive Skin

How do you tell if patients have sensitive skin? The easiest way is to ask them how sensitive their skin is to skin care products, makeup, and soaps. This will usually give you a good idea of their tolerance to topical products.

1. The patient should start by using a pea-sized dab of retinoic acid 0.25% cream at bedtime. The retinoic acid should be applied 20 minutes after gently washing the face with lukewarm water and a mild soap (Purpose, Dove, Neutrogena) or nonsoap cleanser (Cetaphil, Aquanil, SFC). It is dabbed onto the forehead, nose, cheeks, and chin, then gently massaged into the skin. Care should be taken to avoid the oral commissures, orbital canthi, and alar creases, since these areas are easily irritated. Initially, the retinoic acid should not be applied to the lower eyelid, and the applications should stop at the orbital rim. Although no retinoic acid is applied to the lower eyelid, some of it will migrate or smear there during sleep. This small amount allows the sensitive skin of the lower eyelid time to acclimate more gradually than the rest of the face. Gradually, the retinoic acid can be applied closer and closer to the eyelid margin until it is within 2 to 3 mm of the lid margin.

2. If the patient tolerates this strength of retinoic acid without persistent erythema, peeling, or irritation, the strength can be increased to 0.05% cream when the first tube is finished. Later, the strength can be increased to 0.1% cream if needed and tolerated.

3. If, on the other hand, the patient has persistent irritation with the use of retinoic acid 0.025% cream, it can be diluted. This is done by mixing an equal pea-sized dab of retinoic acid with a pea-sized dab of a fragrance-free moisturizer and applying this mixture (now with a concentration of 0.0125%) every night at bedtime. If this is still too irritating, one dab of retinoic acid can be mixed with two dabs of moisturizer, creating a mixture with a retinoic acid concentration of 0.008%.

4. Some physicians have their patients mix the retinoic acid with a topical corticosteroid cream to decrease inflammation. There is some evidence that retinoic acid can prevent the atrophic effects of chronic steroid use. However, there is no evidence that retinoic acid can prevent the formation of telangiectasia associated with chronic topical corticosteroid use. In addition, some evidence suggests that chronic retinoic acid use alone can induce telangiectasia. Therefore, it seems prudent to use the topical steroid only for short periods.

Another option of an antiinflammatory product is Catrix cream. This nonprescription product contains a naturally occurring antiinflammatory agent, a mucopolysaccharide derived from bovine tracheal cartilage. This product decreases the erythema and irritation associated with retinoic acid use. In my experience, its antiinflammatory effects are at least equal to 1% hydrocortisone. However, unlike topical corticosteroids, it does not create atrophy or telangiectasia. Therefore, chronic use of this product is not contraindicated.

I often advocate this product either mixed with retinoic acid at bedtime or applied to the face 5 to 10 minutes after applying retinoic acid. If the patient has marked inflammation, I have them apply this product (available with a sunscreen) each morning as well.

Aggressive Retinoic Acid Use

Patients who have used retinoic acid in the past without problems or those who tell you they have "tough skin" do not need to begin therapy on very low-dose retinoic acid. As a general rule, I start these patients on retinoic acid 0.05% cream at bedtime. The amount applied (pea-sized dab) is the same as in patients with sensitive skin. However, these patients can apply the retinoic acid immediately after washing their face, without waiting 20 minutes. (The skin is usually a little more sensitive immediately after having been washed.)

If patients tolerate 0.05% cream easily and without any initial dermatitis, you can rapidly move them to the 0.1% cream at bedtime. If they tolerate this strength well, you have a few options as to what you can do to increase the effect of the retinoic acid:

1. You can put them on retinoic acid 0.05% liquid. Although this product is highly effective in treating acne, it can be quite drying. I am not convinced that, despite its increased potential for irritation, it is more effective in the treatment of photodamaged skin.
2. You can have them apply the retinoic acid in the morning as well as at bedtime. This may not be a problem for patients who have minimal sun exposure during the day, but it is difficult for patients who are outdoors a lot.
3. You can have them pretreat their skin with a chemical that will enhance the penetration of retinoic acid before applying it. This includes using a cleanser containing salicylic acid (SalAc, Neutrogena Acne Cleanser with salicylic acid) or alpha hydroxy acid (brand names too numerous too mention). The use of topical abrasive scrubs or masks may also enhance the penetration of retinoic acid by thinning the stratum corneum.

Be sure to caution all patients using retinoic acid that their skin will usually be more sensitive to *anything* that would normally irritate it. It is common to see retinoic acid patients with significant irritation from the use of

▶ facial chemical depilatories
▶ hair dye
▶ hair permanents or straighteners
▶ facial waxing

It is safest to avoid these products or to discontinue the application of retinoic acid for 5 to 7 days before using them.

▷ Alpha Hydroxy Acids

Alpha hydroxy acids (AHAs) are a group of organic acids that have recently become popular in the treatment of a variety of skin conditions, particularly those characterized by hyperkeratinization. Several of these acids are derived from fruits, so they are often referred to as "fruit acids." For example, glycolic acid is derived from sugar cane, citric acid from citrus fruit, and malic from apples. Although the concept of a natural fruit acid has been exploited by the lay press, it is important that we realize that the glycolic acid available for use on our patients is created in a laboratory and is not squeezed from fruit.

The exact mechanism of action of AHAs is not completely understood. However, it appears that these acids exert specific, separate effects on the epidermis and the dermis. In the epidermis, the effect is at the level of the stratum granulosum. AHAs create keratinocyte dyscohesion (an "ungluing" of cells), which causes pathologically sticky cells to become loose, allowing them to be shed. This corrects an abnormally thickened stratum corneum, an effect that can persist for up to 14 days after cessation of therapy. This effect is distinctly different than that of other acids, which have a dissolving effect on only the most superficial cells of the stratum corneum. In addition, daily use of AHAs increases epidermal thickness. One small study by Piacquadio and colleagues even showed some reduction in actinic keratoses with daily AHA use.

The dermal effects of AHAs that have been histologically demonstrated are an increase in the deposition of collagen and glycosaminoglycans in the dermis. These effects lead to a thickening of the dermis. Presumably this increase in dermal volume creates the reduction in wrinkles and scars often seen in patients using AHAs.

These dermal changes can be seen without any evidence of inflammation. This supports the concept that there may be a specific direct effect of glycolic acid on the skin that is different from a nonspecific irritant effect. Moy has presented data showing that fibroblast cultures incubated with glycolic acid produce 10 times the amount of hydroxyproline as fibroblasts incubated with normal saline. (Hydroxyproline is a precursor to collagen.)

Several companies manufacture AHA products. Most use glycolic acid, although products containing lactic acid and citric acid are also available. There have been no published studies comparing the relative efficacy of these different alpha hydroxy acids. The question of the effectiveness of varying degrees of neutralization of AHA products is also an important one. Unfortunately, only minimal data about this question are available, despite the claims made by certain companies offering AHA products.

In one small study examining the effect of neutralization on glycolic acid products, it was shown that solutions containing 10% free glycolic acid were

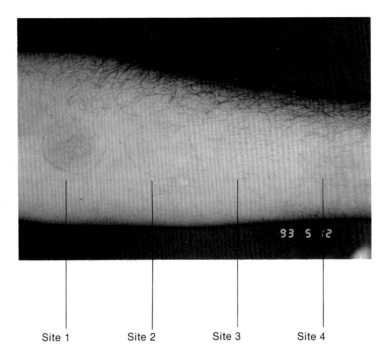

Figure 3-1

Inflammation and scaling induced by 35 days of twice-daily application of 10% free glycolic acid (site 1) and 10% totally neutralized glycolic acid (site 4). This is contrasted with the normal clinical appearance of site 2, which was treated with 10% partially neutralized glycolic acid. Site 3 is a control area treated with no glycolic acid.

Site 1   Site 2   Site 3   Site 4

clinically irritating and caused some reactive hyperkeratosis. Solutions containing 10% glycolic acid that was totally neutralized with sodium hydroxide were also irritating but to a significantly lesser degree than those containing only the free acid. Partially neutralized 10% glycolic acid was well tolerated and showed some of the beneficial epidermal and dermal changes previously documented with AHA use (Fig. 3-1). Therefore, I encourage the use of partially neutralized glycolic acid products, since they appear to be both well tolerated and effective.

It is also important to consider bioavailability, since the absorption of an active compound can be markedly influenced by the chemical composition of the base it is mixed in. Therefore, having a chemist put 10% glycolic acid in an ordinary face cream will not necessarily create as effective a 10% glycolic acid cream as one available from a company experienced in creating and compounding AHA products. My experience with these "homemade" products has been disappointing, suggesting this concept to be true.

More than 70 companies sell AHA products ranging in concentrations from 1% to 30% in the United States. Many are now selling products with slight alterations of the AHA molecules (eg, esterification or polymerization), but no data have been published to suggest that these variants are any better than unadulterated AHAs. For that matter, no data show that these products are even as effective as unadulterated AHAs.

Therefore, it seems prudent to stick to unadulterated AHA products, since they have at least some research supporting their efficacy.

Using Glycolic Acid Products

No one really knows the best way to use glycolic acid products. Normally, when we use an active topical agent to treat a patient's skin, considerable research is available to indicate the most efficacious concentrations, application schedules, and durations of therapy. Unfortunately, no such research exists to help us with AHAs.

The AHAs came on the market at an unusual time. Preliminary data by Drs. Van Scott and Yu show that AHAs can create some changes in the structure of the skin. According to US Food and Drug Administration rules, this would classify AHAs as drugs. If drugs, they have to be appropriately tested before being released to the public. This is a long and expensive process that most companies would prefer to avoid. Rather than subject their AHA products to pharmaceutical testing, many companies put them on the market without making drug claims (eg, "this product removes wrinkles"). Instead, they are advertised as "improving the appearance of fine wrinkles." None of the companies sponsor clinical research because if they prove a product works, it becomes a drug!

It is important to keep in mind that **the reason the AHA products are so popular is that patients like them.** Most people who use AHA products notice improvement in their skin. It may be only a softening of rough skin or it may include improved skin color and wrinkle reduction. Whatever the results, something has changed in the skin; it is not a placebo effect.

Since we really don't know what regimens work best based on research, we are forced to base our decisions on data accumulated from clinical use by patients over the years. In the following box, I present my recommendations for using AHA products based on 5 years of clinical experience.

Key POINTS TO USING AHA PRODUCTS

1. All AHA products may create transient stinging when first applied to the skin. This is normal and not a cause for concern. Persistent stinging, longer than 30 to 60 seconds, implies too strong a product for the patient's skin (the AHA concentration may be too high, or the PH of the product may be too low).
2. AHA products are available in many forms—including cleansers, astringents, creams, lotions, and gels—so it is easy to select the type of product the patient would prefer to use. For example, oily-skinned patients prone to acne usually prefer an astringent or gel rather than a cream. Let the patient tell you what type of product he or she wants to use.
3. It is best to start the patient on low-level products and gradually increase the concentration of the products, rather than to start out on a high strength that may cause irritation. The worst thing you can do is to irritate the skin. This destroys the patient's motivation to continue use of the product.

4. If the patient is currently using retinoic acid without problems, continue its use at bedtime, but add an AHA product in the morning. Again, start with a low-concentration product initially.

5. The AHA products rarely cause an increase in photosensitivity, but patients should be cautioned to wear a broad-spectrum sunscreen each morning to protect their newly improved skin.

6. Patients using AHAs usually build up a tolerance to any irritation they may initially experience. Research has shown that using 12% lactic acid salt (Lac-Hydrin) for several weeks causes the skin to become less reactive to an irritant, sodium lauryl sulfate, than skin untreated with lactic acid.

Almost all patients can tolerate an 8% to 10% AHA product to start with. If a patient has a history of very sensitive skin, I may start with a 4% glycolic acid cream (Avon's ANEW) or 5% lactic acid (Penecare, Lac-Hydrin 5) once daily and increase it to twice daily after several days if there is no evidence of irritation.

For patients with normal skin, start with a product they can use easily. If they are using night cream, substitute a cream that contains AHAs. If they do not like to wear any lotions, creams, or gels, start them on an AHA cleanser or astringent once or twice a day. Because most patients interested in AHA products have photoaged skin, they often have some type of dyschromias with hyperpigmented lesions. These patients do extremely well on a combination of AHA mixed with hydroquinone or kojic acid (NeoStrata's AHA gel for spots and skin lightening, or Physician's Choice of Arizona's pigment gel). These combination products are available only in a gel form. It dries rapidly, however, and most patients will apply it, wait a few minutes for it to dry, then apply a sunscreen in the morning or a moisturizer at night.

Once patients use their initial products for 6 to 8 weeks, they should be reexamined. If they are tolerating the products well and are showing signs of clinical improvement, you may elect not to change the regimen. If they are tolerating the products but showing minimal or no clinical improvement, you need to make the regimen more aggressive. This is usually done by following one or more of these suggestions:

▶ Increasing the concentration of glycolic acid to 12% to 15% twice a day
▶ Adding retinoic acid at bedtime to the regimen (see next section on combined retinoic acid and AHA therapy)
▶ Adding an AHA cleanser or astringent twice a day before applying the cream, lotion, or gel

▶ Adding a 20% or 30% glycolic acid cream (Glytone, Veritas) for 30 minutes up to 8 hours one or two nights a week. The product is left on the skin until it causes persistent stinging, then washed off. This type of take-home "minipeel" usually induces some mild flaking for 1 or 2 days. *Be cautious,* this strength glycolic acid can cause serious burns if left on the skin too long. Only prescribe these 20% to 30% products for patients who understand how to use them.

▶ Trying a series of glycolic acid peels (discussed in the section on AHA peels)

Although most patients show skin improvement on a regimen of AHAs, the degree of improvement may not be sufficient (even with AHA peels). In these cases, the use of more aggressive peeling agents may be needed to achieve the desired results. However, because AHA products and peels have such low morbidity, it is reasonable to try them before moving to more aggressive treatments with higher morbidity.

What Brands of Alpha Hydroxy Acid Products Do I Recommend?

I don't want to endorse any particular company, but there are a few that have been making AHA products for years and have a good track record. I have seen improvement in thousands of patients using these brands of products. (This is not to imply that other companies do not make good products, I just don't have extensive experience with them.)

The products I use are as follows:

Penecare by Penederm—lactic acid 5% and 7.5%

NeoStrata—glycolic acid 8% to 15%; one product with hydroquinone (this company is partly owned by Drs. Van Scott and Yu)

Therapeutic Dermatologic Formula by Dermatologic Cosmetic Labs—glycolic acid 8% to 20%; one product with hydroquinone

Glytone by C&M Pharmacal—glycolic acid 5% to 30%

Physician's Choice of Arizona—various products containing a blend of AHAs, with and without hydroquinone and kojic acid

MD Formulations by Herald Pharmacal—glycolic acid 4% to 18%

Aqua Glycolic by Herald Pharmacal—glycolic acid 10% to 12%

Veritas by Dermatologic Skin Care Laboratory—glycolic acid 8% to 30%

▷ Combination Therapy

Studies have shown that retinoic acid and AHAs can create similar histologic changes in the skin, including

- ▶ a thinner stratum corneum
- ▶ a thicker epidermis
- ▶ increased glycosaminoglycan deposition
- ▶ increased collagen deposition

If retinoic acid and AHAs work on different receptors in the cells, a combination of both products would have the possibility of giving a more marked histologic change than either product alone.

During the past few years an ever-increasing number of patients have been using combinations of retinoic acid and AHA creams as part of their daily maintenance programs. I have thought for several years that this type of combination therapy is more effective than using either product alone (Fig. 3-2). It also gives the physician the ability to maximize patient benefits while limiting side effects, since lower concentrations of each product can be used if they work synergistically.

In 1993, an article by Kligman documented what many of us believed—namely, that retinoic acid and glycolic acid can be used together safely and with no real increase in the irritation of the skin. It is even possible that long-term use

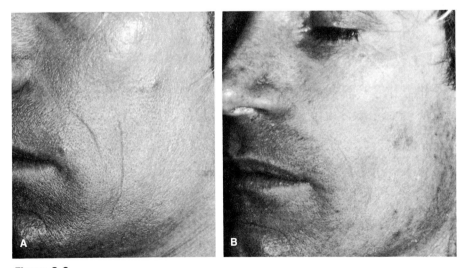

Figure 3-2
(*A*) Wrinkles in a patient who used 0.1% retinoic acid cream twice a day for 1 year. (*B*) The same patient 6 months after adding 10% glycolic acid lotion twice daily to his daily regimen. A dramatic improvement in wrinkles is seen.

of glycolic acid may decrease the skin's ability to become irritated, thereby allowing the addition of retinoic acid to the daily regimen. In 1992, Lavker and coworkers demonstrated that the use of 12% ammonium lactate (Lac-Hydrin) twice daily for 2 weeks decreased the skin's reaction to a known irritant, sodium laurel sulfate. Granted, this study was performed with lactic acid, not glycolic acid, but these two AHAs appear to have similar effects. It seems reasonable to assume that glycolic acid may decrease the skin's reactivity as well. My clinical experience suggests this is true. Therefore, when using retinoic acid and glycolic acid creams on the same patient, start the glycolic acid product first; then, after 2 weeks of AHA use, add retinoic acid.

Because there was a suggestion of a synergistic effect with retinoic acid and AHAs, Dr. Steve Hoefflin and I undertook a study to examine the histologic effects of the combined use of these two products. On one side of the face, patients used retinoic acid 0.05% to 0.1% cream at bedtime and 15% glycolic acid gel in the morning; on the other, they used only retinoic acid 0.05% to 0.1% cream at bedtime. Biopsy samples from each treatment site were taken after 4 to 8 weeks of therapy, and the two treatment regimens were compared. The skin treated with both retinoic acid and glycolic acid showed a thicker epidermis and more glycosaminoglycan deposition in the dermis than the skin treated with retinoic acid alone. The difference was more striking in some patients than others (Fig. 3-3) but was seen in all five patients. As expected, no new collagen deposition was seen in any patient, since this was a short-term study (new collagen deposition is reportedly seen only after months of retinoic acid or AHA use). A larger long-term study is underway. With all this information, it certainly seems reasonable to attempt to use both products as part of a treatment regimen for patients who desire the best possible response.

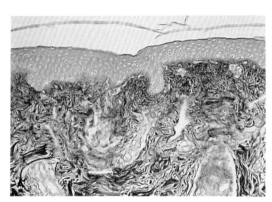 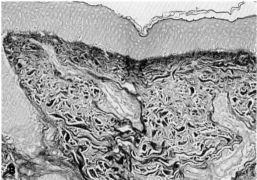

Figure 3-3

(*A*) Preauricular skin in a patient after 6 weeks of using 0.05% retinoic acid cream at bedtime. (*B*) Preauricular skin of the same patient after 6 weeks of using 0.05% retinoic acid cream every night and 15% gycolic acid gel every morning. There is an increase in epidermal thickness and glycosaminoglycans deposition in the dermis (seen as blue-staining material with Hales stain).

There are several key points to keep in mind when designing a combination regimen for your patient:

Do not mix retinoic acid cream and AHA cream together. No one has examined whether mixing retinoic acid and AHA creams together creates a product that is clinically effective. It may be possible that the mixture becomes "inactivated" or the diffusion coefficient is significantly altered, preventing the active ingredients from penetrating into the skin. Therefore, it is best to do one of the following:

  ▶ Use retinoic acid at bedtime and AHA in the morning.
  ▶ Use the AHA twice a day and the retinoic acid only at night, but wait for 1 hour after the nighttime AHA treatment before applying retinoic acid.
  ▶ Use a twice-daily AHA product with a base that is a solution or gel so it penetrates rapidly into the skin. Apply this product and wait until it dries fully (5 to 10 minutes), then apply retinoic acid at bedtime.

Always start with low-concentration products first, then increase their concentration over time. Because both retinoic acid and AHAs increase the penetration of other chemicals used on the skin, it appears that lower doses of both products give results comparable to high doses of either product alone, but with decreased potential side effects.

If the patient has a red, ruddy complexion or has dilated facial capillaries, minimize retinoic acid use. Most physicians believe that long-term retinoic acid use can increase facial telangiectasia. At this time, no evidence indicates that long-term AHA use creates a similar effect. Therefore, in patients at risk for facial erythema and telangiectasia, it is prudent to use little or no retinoic acid and to use a more aggressive regimen of AHAs.

If the patient has problems with photosensitivity and retinoic acid use, minimize retinoic acid use. Some patients who spend a great deal of time outdoors may complain about photosensitivity with retinoic acid use, even if they wear a daily sunscreen. In these patients, lowering the retinoic acid's concentration or even discontinuing its use while increasing the concentration of AHA products may still provide clinical improvement, but with much less photoreactivity.

Select the appropriate vehicle (base) for each patient's skin. For any long-term topical therapy to be effective, patients must be willing to use the products long-term. If a patient has dry skin and you give him or her products in a drying vehicle (like a solution or some gels), the skin will become drier and probably irritated. Conversely, if a patient has thick, oily skin and you give him or her two or three creams to apply each day, the skin will feel greasy and the patient may not to want to use the products. Therefore, be sure to select the appropriate vehicle for each patient.

Once the patient is on a daily regimen with both products, the skin must be allowed time to improve. Most patients will begin to notice

- ▶ improvement in skin texture within 2 to 3 weeks
- ▶ reduction of pore size in 3 to 6 weeks
- ▶ improvement in mottled pigmentation in 6 to 12 weeks
- ▶ improvement in wrinkles in 8 to 24 weeks

If a patient is tolerating the regimen well and getting significant clinical improvement, there is no need to change it. If, on the other hand, a patient shows little improvement, the regimen needs to be more aggressive. Usually, the easiest way to increase a regimen is to increase the concentration of AHA first. Because most people tolerate AHAs better than retinoic acid, it makes sense to increase these products first. This allows the patient to have the potential for better results with a decreased risk of side effects. If the patient can tolerate an increased concentration of AHAs but still fails to improve much, the next step would be to increase the concentration of retinoic acid. This constant upward adjustment of concentrations allows you to maximize the patient's benefits.

After 6 months or so, most patients have reached a plateau of improvement. If their results are acceptable to both of you, they should stay on maintenance therapy. Maintenance therapy does not have to be as aggressive as the initial therapy. If patients are comfortable with their daily regimen, I think it is best to leave them on it (now an ingrained habit). If they have some level of irritation with their regimen, I would decrease the concentration of one or both products to allow them to maintain improvement without side effects.

At this time, we know that using retinoic acid once or twice a week maintains the histologic improvement achieved from long-term daily retinoic acid use. However, we do not know whether the same is true for AHAs. Thus, it is best to maintain daily use of AHA products but to decrease the concentration if the patient experiences irritation.

▷ Other Nonpeel Methods

With the popularity of retinoic acid and AHAs for skin rejuvenation, there has been an ever-increasing demand to know how these products work. Many people have hypothesized that these products are irritants that induce increased cellular turnover. Those who disagree state that although patients have histologic evidence of increased cellular turnover, they do not always show evidence of irritation (inflammation).

In 1989, Wilhelm and colleagues showed that the daily application of a known chemical irritant, sodium lauryl sulfate, to the skin of the volar forearm created about a 50% reduction in the turnover time of the stratum corneum compared with the turnover time of skin treated with water. This is rather strong evidence that mitotic activity can be increased by daily applications of an irritant before there is clinical evidence of inflammation. However, all patients exhibited clinical evidence of inflammation within 10 days of using the product. This reaction is not seen in patients using AHAs or low-dose retinoic acid, who may show histologic evidence of increased cellular growth without any clinical evidence of inflammation during months of use.

A study by Marks and associates compared the histologic effects of retinoic acid on photodamaged skin of the forearm with the histologic effects of similar skin treated with an abrasive agent. Biopsy specimens from both treatment areas failed to show any significant inflammation. However, they did demonstrate similar effects of increased epidermal thickness and increased keratinocyte production. The productive question raised by this study is whether these histologic changes, previously attributed to retinoic acid, are nonspecific effects that can be replicated with irritants or abrasives.

On a less scientific note, does it really matter what the mechanism of action is? Obviously, understanding the true mechanism of action is important so that better therapies can be devised in the future, but until that time . . . If photodamage can be improved by any of these nonpeel methods, we should be happy that we have several possible topical therapies at our disposal.

Manual of Chemical Peels: Superficial and Medium Depth, by Mark G. Rubin.
J.B. Lippincott Company, Philadelphia, © 1995.

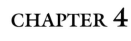

CHAPTER **4**

BASIC CONCEPTS IN SKIN PEELING

Pharmaceutical Considerations ▶ *Priming* ▶
Wound Healing ▶ *Regional Peels* ▶
Repeeling ▶ *Anesthesia* ▶ *The Difference
Between Facial and Nonfacial Skin Peels*

All chemical peels are based on the same premise—the application of a cauterant or escharotic agent to the skin, with the creation of some type of wound. Although there are many peeling agents and many variations in their use, several basic concepts apply to all types of peels.

This chapter considers basic, fundamental concepts in skin peeling. You must have a strong grasp of these concepts to become proficient in performing peels.

▷ Pharmaceutical Considerations
James Dolezal, MD

To provide peel results that are reproducible, as many variables as possible should be standardized. Variation of factors such as skin type and biologic response is inevitable in peels. Techniques such as method and pressure of application often vary from operator to operator, but with training, such variation can be minimized. Anomalies in the preparation itself, normally considered a nonvariable within any given strength, are a source of significant variation.

The outstanding performance of our drug industry in providing quality pharmaceuticals has resulted in physicians' near complete acceptance of a drug's quantitative and qualitative attributes. A physician's drug decisions involve consideration of the appropriateness of a chemical compound for the condition to be treated. The physician chooses a chemical compound then decides on the dose and dosage form. Normally, little to no consideration is required about the actual manufacture of the preparation.

Legal Standards

When chemicals are used in preparations intended for use as a drug or medicament, USP grade material should be used. The initials *USP* after a drug or chemical name indicates that the material so labeled meets the standards of the United States Pharmacopoeia. The USP is a compendium that provides a legal standard for the identity, purity, strength, and quality of listed drugs. A complete revision of the USP is issued once every 5 years, with interim supplements. The current edition is USP XXII. Both active and inactive ingredients are considered important. For drugs not listed in the USP, other compendiums can serve as a supplemental source to provide a legal standard of purity, such as the National Formulary (NF) and British Pharmacopoeia (BP). When a previously listed drug is no longer listed in the USP, the last USP edition to include the drug or ingredient may also serve as a standard. In that event, material meeting the standards of that USP could be referred to as such, or simply labeled USP and modified by the appropriate edition number, for example, USP XVIII. Drugs meeting the standards of these compendiums are considered medical grade.

The accessibility of skin lends itself to experimentation. Chemicals that have not previously been considered as medical—and so not subjected to tests for medical purity, quality, identity and strength—may be studied and reports given on beneficial properties. Such accounts may result in relatively widespread use. Examples of such are azelaic acid, kojic acid, glycolic acid, pyruvic acid, dinitrochlorobenzene, and diphenylcyclopropanone. These compounds can be obtained in industrial, laboratory, reagent, or technical grades. Such grades have not been evaluated or processed with consideration of their suitability for use as drugs. If a chemical is not listed in any official medical compendium, chemical manufacturers can define standards of purity for the chemical for use in cosmetic products. When the chemical meets these standards, it can then be called "cosmetic grade."

▷ Priming

Preparing the skin for a peel, or priming it, is one of the most important concepts in chemical rejuvenation. The goals of skin preparation are as follows.

Reduce wound healing time. The use of retinoic acid 0.1% cream daily for at least 2 weeks before a 35% trichloroacetic acid (TCA) facial peel speeds reepithelization by about 24 hours. Similar results are seen with pretreating the skin of the forearm before a peel. Obviously, the faster the skin reepithelializes, the less risk of developing an area of accidental premature peeling or infection.

It is not known whether using an alpha hydroxy acid (AHA) cream before a TCA peel speeds reepithelization in the same manner retinoic acid does. In my own practice, I have not noticed any significant delayed healing in patients undergoing TCA peels if they were primed with AHA rather than retinoic acid.

Allow for more uniform penetration of the peeling agent. Our "living skin" is protected by the stratum corneum, which functions as a protective barrier. The thickness of the stratum corneum varies in different areas of the face. Therefore, its ability to block the penetration of a peeling agent also varies throughout the face.

Thinning the stratum corneum allows better penetration of the peeling agent. This can be achieved with the daily use of retinoic acid or AHA products. In addition, mechanical abrasion of the skin with gauze pads just before the peel serves to thin or even remove the stratum corneum.

Decrease the risk of postinflammatory hyperpigmentation. Any peel capable of producing inflammation is able to induce postinflammatory hyperpigmentation. Contrary to common belief, this reaction is not that uncommon in Caucasians, although its incidence is greater in patients of Asian, Hispanic, or African American heritage.

Both retinoic acid and glycolic acid have been shown to have a skin-lightening effect by enhancing the dispersion of melanin granules throughout the epidermis. This effect appears to be mildly helpful in reducing the incidence of postinflammatory hyperpigmentation.

The use of bleaching agents such as hydroquinone, kojic acid, and azelaic acid can have a significant impact on the prevention of postinflammatory hyperpigmentation. Remember, these bleaching agents are not true bleachers. They work by inhibiting tyrosinase, the enzyme responsible for the conversion of tyrosine to L-dopa. Therefore, using a tyrosinase-blocking agent for several weeks before a peel may actually decrease the skin's ability to create melanin, thereby making it more difficult for the hyperpigmentation reaction to occur. No one has examined the exact length of time these products need to be used prior to the peel to achieve the best results. The general rule is to start using these products along with retinoic acid or an AHA at least 2 weeks before the peel.

Enforce the concept of a maintenance regimen and determine which products the patient's skin tolerates. All patients should use some form of maintenance therapy after their peels to achieve and maintain the best results. After a chemical peel, the skin is more sensitive for a few days to a few weeks, depending on the depth of the peel. Therefore, it is not uncommon for some patients to experience erythema, scaling, or irritation from the use of certain products in the immediate postpeel phase. It is difficult, if not impossible, to differentiate a specific allergic sensitivity due to a certain product from a short-term irritant sensitivity limited to the immediate postpeel time frame.

Starting all patients before peeling on the products they will use as part of their postpeel maintenance programs allows you to determine which products their skin tolerates when in a normal, noninflamed state. For example, if before the peel, a patient can easily tolerate retinoic acid 0.05% cream at bedtime and Shade UVA Guard sunscreen in the morning, but these same products create irritation in the immediate postpeel phase, it would be safe to assume that the patient is having a temporary sensitivity secondary to the peel that should subside within a few days rather than a chronic allergic reaction to these products. This concept is especially important with respect to sunscreens, since many patients are irritated by certain sunscreens.

Consider the example of a postpeel patient with postinflammatory hyperpigmentation who experiences erythema and burning after beginning therapy for the first time with retinoic acid, hydroquinone, and a sunscreen. In this unpleasant situation, you don't know which product is to blame for the reaction and you don't want to stop them all and allow the hyperpigmentation to continue.

Establish patient compliance and eliminate inappropriate patients. The use of a prepeel regimen demands the daily application of certain products. If it is an aggressive regimen, it may initially create some mild erythema or scaling.

If a patient is unable to stick to his or her daily regimen or if he or she is extremely unhappy with the side effects initially associated with it, this patient may not be a good candidate for a peel. Remember, the best results obtained with a peel depend on daily skin care before, during, and after the peel. If a patient is unable to stick to a daily regimen for a few weeks before a peel, you should have serious doubts about his or her ability to follow your recommended regimen during and after the peel. In addition, a patient who complains a great deal about mild erythema or scaling during the prepeel phase is highly likely to be much more unhappy with the erythema and scaling associated with the postpeel phase.

Always keep in mind that a poorly compliant patient can ruin a good peel by creating complications. **If you have any doubt about a patient's level of motivation or ability to follow your instructions, don't perform the peel!**

Method

Now that you understand the concept of priming the skin, how do you go about doing it? The basic regimen is very simple and is adjusted slightly for each patient.

Agents commonly used to prime the skin for peels include

- ▶ retinoic acid
- ▶ AHAs
- ▶ hydroquinone
- ▶ kojic acid
- ▶ broad-spectrum sunscreen

Since you need to stimulate epidermal cell growth and thin the stratum corneum, you can use retinoic acid or AHA. Both of these products can fulfill these two criteria. As mentioned, we know retinoic acid speeds reepithelialization, but we do not know whether this is true for AHAs. Therefore, if you are going to do a medium depth peel, which takes 5 to 7 days to heal, it is beneficial to prime the patient with retinoic acid to speed healing. In a patient undergoing a 3- or 4-day superficial peel, the effect of retinoic acid on the speed of healing is of less significance.

Certainly, if the patient has very sensitive skin, a ruddy complexion with telangiectasia, or extreme sun exposure, it is advantageous to use AHAs rather than retinoic acid to prime the patient. AHAs would be much better tolerated by the patient. On the other hand, in a patient with thick, oily skin, you may want to use retinoic acid at night and an AHA in the morning to get the best priming effects possible.

The minimum amount of time allowable to sufficiently prime a patient is 2 weeks. Most physicians believe that a period of 4 to 6 weeks gives an even better effect. The important thing to remember is that you need a minimum of 2 weeks. **Do not perform peels on skin that is not primed appropriately.**

What concentration retinoic acid or AHA do you need to use? This varies from one patient to the next. The idea is to get enough active drug into the skin to achieve the effect you want without creating a dermatitis. If you induce a dermatitis and then perform a peel on the skin when it is inflamed, the resulting peel will inadvertently be deeper. Therefore, it is best to start with the lower strength retinoic acid or AHA creams and increase their concentration if the patient tolerates it well (see Chapter 3). This is one of the reasons that it is helpful to have more than 2 weeks before the peel to establish an appropriate priming routine. Remember, **if a patient presents to your office on the day of his or her peel with a severe facial dermatitis you should not perform the peel.** It is much safer to discontinue the priming regimen or to decrease its concentration and to perform the peel later when the patient has stabilized. Although the patient may be unhappy with such a schedule disruption, it is safer to postpone the peel than to create an accidental deep peel with potential complications.

In addition to starting patients on retinoic acid, AHAs, or both, you also need to have them on a daily broad-spectrum sunscreen every morning as well as some type of gentle cleanser. For sunscreens, I like to use Shade UVA Guard, Durascreen, Ti-Screen Natural, or Neutrogena chemical-free sunscreen. There are many choices of mild, nonirritating cleansers; I recommend Purpose soap or Neutrogena regular soap. If the patient likes a mild liquid cleanser rather than bar soap, I recommend Cetaphil, Aquanil, or SFC.

Priming Patients With Dyschromias

Every patient undergoing a peel (of any depth) to improve hyperpigmentation needs to be on a bleaching agent before the peel. This is also true for any patient at risk for developing postinflammatory hyperpigmentation. (Remember to ask patients whether they experience hyperpigmentation from trauma, and then examine their skin for signs of postinflammatory hyperpigmentation.)

The most commonly used bleaching agents are hydroquinone and kojic acid. These agents are not really bleachers; they block the conversion of tyrosine to L-dopa, thereby decreasing the melanocyte's ability to create new melanin. (A true bleaching agent would create immediate lightening of existing melanin.) Priming the skin with one of these products before the peel seems to significantly reduce the incidence of dyschromia after a peel. No one has studied how long these products need to be used before a peel to create the optimal effect. Most physicians start them at the same time they start retinoic acid or AHA.

The choice of hydroquinone products includes

- ▶ 3% hydroquinone in a hydroalcoholic base (Melanex, Neutrogena Dermatologics)
- ▶ 4% hydroquinone in a cream base (Eldoquine Forte, ICN Pharmaceuticals)
- ▶ 4% hydroquinone with a chemical-free sunblock in a cream base (Eldopaque, ICN Pharmaceuticals)
- ▶ 4% hydroquinone with a chemical sunscreen in a cream or gel base (Solaquin Forte, ICN Pharmaceuticals)
- ▶ 2% hydroquinone with 10% glycolic acid in a gel base (NeoStrata Gel for Age Spots and Skin Lightening, NeoStrata)
- ▶ 2% hydroquinone and 2% kojic acid with 6% AHA in a gel base (Pigment Gel, Physician's Choice of Arizona)

Although the last two products listed have only 2% hydroquinone (the same concentration sold in nonprescription products), they are at least as efficacious as the prescription strength 4% hydroquinone products. Actually, several studies show that they are more effective bleachers than the 4% hydroquinone products listed. Some patients with very sensitive or dry skin may prefer a cream-based hydroquinone, but most patients tolerate a gel well. In addition, the gels are well accepted because they rapidly absorb into the skin and can be followed by the application of moisturizer, sunscreen, or makeup.

The only kojic acid products for sale in the United States at this time are made by Physician's Choice of Arizona. This company makes several gels containing kojic acid 2% to 3% with and without hydroquinone, all in an AHA gel base. These products are especially helpful for patients who cannot tolerate hydroquinone. The only other bleaching agent for hydroquinone-sensitive patients is azelaic acid, which is irritating to most patients. In addition, azelaic acid has not been a very effective bleaching agent in my experience, and it takes 4 to 6 months to achieve its maximum response.

Many physicians routinely prime all of their prepeel patients with a bleaching agent in an effort to decrease the risk of postinflammatory hyperpigmentation. This is an acceptable routine since the products are usually well tolerated (with the exception of azelaic acid). There are reports of permanent hyperpigmentation or acquired ochronosis due to prolonged use of hydroquinones (particularly at high strengths). This has been reported in several black patients and in a few Asian or Hispanic patients. I am unaware of any reports of this condition in Caucasian patients.

If you are concerned about long-term use of bleaching agents, patients can safely stop using them 2 to 3 months after a peel. Unfortunately, some patients may experience a gradual recurrence of hyperpigmentation if they discontinue use of bleaching agents. If this occurs, the patients usually respond well to resumption of their bleaching regimen.

▷ Wound Healing

When the skin reepithelializes from any wound, including a skin peel, it does so by the lateral migration of epithelial cells from pilosebaceous units. It is the peeler's goal to create an environment conducive to the rapid migration of these cells, thereby accelerating the wound healing.

It seems that every physician has a favorite regimen for the treatment of wounded, peeling skin. Some advocate keeping the skin dry during the healing phase, whereas others like to apply numerous compresses throughout the day, or encourage frequent showering. Still others like to apply copious amounts of ointments or emollients to keep the healing tissue moist.

When it comes to the choice of which topical emollients to use, the number of physician regimens increases dramatically. Part of the confusion comes from the fact that the published studies examining the effect of topical products on wound healing do not use peeling skin as their model. Commonly, postoperative surgical incisional wounds or dermatome-induced wounds in animals are used. These studies have shown that certain commonly used products, such as 3% hydrogen peroxide, 1% povidone-iodine, and 0.5% chlorhexidine, can all delay wound healing. Other studies have shown that wounds kept moist heal faster than wounds allowed to dry out. In addition, Geronemus and associates showed that the base of the "moisturizer" products affected the rate of wound healing. A "water in oil" cream base significantly enhanced healing over a petrolatum-based product in animal models. A clinical study by Elson suggested that petrolatum-treated peels and dermabrasions in humans healed significantly faster than those treated with emollient creams. Because of this information and other conflicting studies, it is difficult to decide what type of base is the most effective in the treatment of peeling skin.

If topical antibiotic ointments are used after a peel, allergic contact dermatitis is a concern. Over 5% of patients treated with a topical antibiotic containing Neomycin have allergic reactions to it. Therefore, it is advisable to avoid products containing Neomycin (ie, Neosporin, Mycitracin, certain generic triple-antibiotic creams).

A multitude of other wound-healing agents have been advocated to treat peeling skin, including aloe vera, vitamin E oil, Preparation H (with skin respiratory factor), A&D ointment, vegetable shortening (Crisco), and Silvadene cream. Vitamin E and aloe vera, however, have also been implicated in cases of allergic contact dermatitis, and Silvadene cream (containing 1% sulfadiazine silver) is contraindicated in patients with known allergies to sulfa drugs. Anecdotally, it appears that peeling patients heal at about the same speed regardless of which product is used.

Certainly, patient comfort is increased if the peeling skin is kept moist with some type of emollient. This decreases itching and tightness of the skin, which helps patients to avoid scratching or touching their skin. The less the skin is manipulated during the healing phase, the lower the chance of complications developing secondary to premature peeling of the skin.

Unfortunately, I don't know which postpeel product is the best to use. I have used all products listed and have found their healing times to be fairly similar. The only product I have used that is an effective antiinflammatory agent as well as an accelerator of wound healing is bovine tracheal cartilage 20% in petrolatum. Unfortunately, the commercially available form of this product (Catrix) is only a 5% concentration and does not appear to be as effective as the 20% strength.

The important concept here is that all levels of peels are chemical burns of the skin. The healing skin needs to be treated with some product to create a good wound-healing environment and to keep the patient comfortable. I believe any bland emollient will fulfill these two functions to some degree. The deeper the peel, the greater the need to use a heavier emollient or an ointment, since deeper peels become very dry as they heal. Failure to adequately moisturize the healing skin can lead to fissuring of the peeling skin with associated irritation, itching, or infection.

▷ Regional Peels

The concept of regional or segmental peels is rarely much of a problem for superficial or medium depth peels. With deep peels, the alteration in skin color and texture makes the results of a regional peel look distinctly different from unpeeled skin (Fig. 4-1). For that reason, regional deep peels are usually performed in areas of cosmetic units. With lighter peels, this is much less of a problem since the degree of change in pigment and texture is much less.

However, patients with significant dyschromias or severe photodamage who undergo regional peels may display an obvious line of demarcation. This can be minimized in the following ways:

1. Feather the peel beyond the border of the area you want to peel. This is usually best done with a slightly weaker peeling solution than that used for the regional peel.
2. Apply bleaching agents, sunscreens, and either AHAs or retinoic acid to the surrounding skin to lighten it and improve its texture.

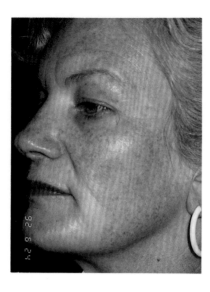

Figure 4-1

Marked hypopigmentation in a patient who had undergone a previous perioral phenol peel.

3. Peel the rest of the face with a very light peeling agent that has no risk and no significant downtime, but that can still give the patient some improvement in skin quality.

▷ Repeeling

Because superficial and medium depth peels are often done repeatedly on the same patient to achieve the best results, the question arises, When is it safe to repeel a patient?

The answer depends on however deep the previous peel was, because that will determine how long it takes the skin to heal from the wound. If you repeel the patient before the skin has had a chance to heal adequately, the second peel will penetrate deeper and increase the risk of complications. The following are general frequency guidelines for safe repeeling, based on the depth of the previous peel:

Very superficial (stratum corneum) peels: These peels can be performed as often as once a week.

Superficial (intraepidermal) peels: These peels can be repeated every 2 to 6 weeks, depending on how much epidermal necrosis is created. A full-thickness epidermal peel should not be repeated for at least 6 weeks, whereas a partial-thickness epidermal peel may be repeated within 2 or 3 weeks.

Medium depth (papillary dermis) peels: These peels can be repeated every 3 to 6 months.

These time frames are approximate. Everyone heals at a different rate, and a complication can significantly slow down healing. A good rule of thumb is **never repeel a patient who has sensitivity or erythema persisting from a previous peel.** These patients are not completely healed from the previous peel, and their response to another peel will be exaggerated.

▷ Anesthesia

The sting or burn associated with a chemical peel is completely different from other types of discomfort a patient may have felt, including a thermal burn. It is a brief, not constant burning, which builds up like a wave of heat. Usually, the burning is at its most severe when the erythema or frost has reached its maximum on the skin. It is important to be truthful and tell patients they will have some discomfort but also to reassure them that it will be brief.

Superficial Peels

As a general rule, anesthesia is unnecessary when performing superficial peels. Although patient tolerance to procedures varies tremendously, I have never seen a patient who required sedatives or analgesics during a superficial intraepidermal peel. The use of a fan and some words of encouragement from you and your assistants is normally all a patient needs. It is important for you to be aware, and to relay to the patient, that the stinging or burning associated with a peel varies with different chemicals (eg, Jessner's solution stings longer than 10% TCA). Thus, if you change peeling agents on subsequent peels for a patient, the peel will feel different. However, all superficial peeling agents create transient discomfort that persists only 15 to 30 minutes at most.

Medium Depth Peels

As the peel penetrates deeper into the skin, the sensation becomes more intense and more uncomfortable. Normally, I do not sedate patients undergoing medium depth peels, but I do encourage them to take two aspirins 30 to 60 minutes before the peel. The aspirin blocks prostaglandins, which help mediate the burning of the peel. In addition, I use a fan to help cool the patient during the peel, and I perform the peel in sections, allowing one section to cool down before proceeding to the next.

Many physicians routinely use analgesics or sedatives for medium depth peels. This allows for a much faster procedure, since it is not necessary to stop partway through the peel to let the patient cool down. However, it also makes the peel more expensive and may increase the chance of a systemic reaction or of gastrointestinal upset. The most commonly used medications with medium depth peels are intramuscular meperidine (Demerol) and hydroxyzine (Vistaril), sublingual diazepam (Valium), and intravenous midazolam (Versed) or fentanyl (Sublimaze).

Another option is the use of nerve blocks before the peel. This can significantly decrease the burning of a medium depth peel, but it takes at least eight separate injections to adequately anesthetize the full face. Many patients would prefer 2 or 3 minutes of moderate burning associated with the peel to numerous facial injections.

As a word of caution, any topical anesthetic that creates vasoconstriction (eg, EMLA) can increase the depth of a TCA peel. Therefore, if you use a topical anesthetic, it is best to use a lower strength of TCA than you were originally planning. Failure to notice this vasoconstriction will lead to an inadvertent deeper peel.

▷ The Difference Between Facial and Nonfacial Skin Peels

When considering peels of nonfacial areas, the first priority is to realize that these areas generally do not heal as well as the face. This is usually the case with surgical excision and cryotherapy, and it is especially true with dermabrasion and peels.

When the skin reepithelializes after a skin peel, it does so by the proliferation of epithelial cells from pilosebaceous units (hair follicles and sebaceous glands), which migrate laterally to cover the denuded areas with a new epidermis (Fig. 4-2). Studies have shown that there are 30 times as many pilosebaceous units on the face as there are on the neck or chest, and 40 times as many as on the dorsal

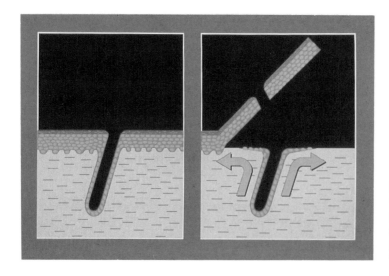

Figure 4-2

The epidermis reepithelizes by the lateral migration of epithelial cells from the pilosebaceous unit (hair follicle).

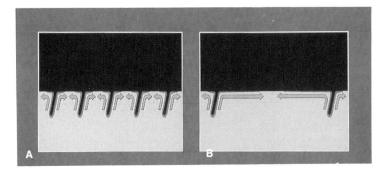

Figure 4-3

Nonfacial wounds (*B*) take longer to reepithelialize than facial wounds (*A*) because there are fewer pilosebaceous units in nonfacial areas.

arms and hands. This means that these nonfacial areas take significantly longer to reepithelialize (Fig. 4-3). The longer it takes a wound to reepithelialize, the greater the risk of a complication.

In addition, certain areas of the body are more prone to hypertrophic scarring. These areas will heal with a poorer-quality scar than other areas that suffered exactly the same type of physical trauma. Therefore, it is prudent not to perform dermal peeling in these areas because of the increased risk of scarring. A familiar example to most of us is the concept of not performing dermabrasion on the chest or back because of the poor cosmetic results usually obtained.

In peeling nonfacial areas, the following rules apply:

1. It usually takes 50% to 100% longer for nonfacial areas to heal than for the face to heal. The patient needs to be sure he or she has the time to undergo this type of therapy before having it done.
2. Since dermal peels on the arms, hands, neck, and chest are more prone to healing with scarring or abnormal textural changes, it is safer to perform epidermal peels in these areas. Therefore, dermal hyperpigmentation and most types of scars on nonfacial areas should not be treated with peeling, since they will not improve significantly.
3. Most nonfacial peels are undertaken to improve fine wrinkling and blotchy discoloration (including age spots). One intraepidermal peel is usually not sufficient to give these patients their best results. Therefore, nonfacial peels are usually repeated several times to achieve the best response.
4. Most nonfacial peels are performed on large areas of skin (a larger surface area than the face). Therefore, if you use a peeling agent with potential toxicity, these patients are at greater risk of developing a systemic reaction. In addition, the larger the area wounded, the more difficult it is for patients to adequately care for it, and the greater the chance of a complication, particularly premature peeling or infections.

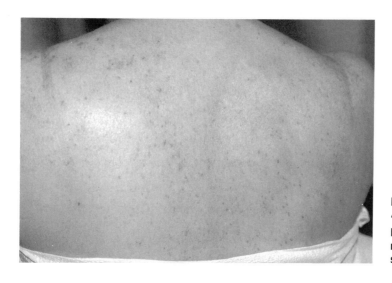

Figure 4-4

"Sunburn freckles" on the back are hyperpigmented macules due to a previous sunburn.

Specific Areas of Nonfacial Peeling

The most common requests for nonfacial peels are as follows:

Back

▶ To remove sunburn freckles across the shoulders and upper back (Fig. 4-4)
▶ To improve acne scars
▶ To improve postinflammatory hyperpigmentation from acne

Chest

▶ To improve hyperpigmented macules, usually lentigines or flat seborrheic keratoses but occasionally sunburn freckles
▶ To improve acne scars, particularly hypopigmented scars in a area of vasodilated and hyperpigmented actinic damage (Fig. 4-5)
▶ To improve postinflammatory hyperpigmentation due to acne
▶ To improve fine wrinkling, often vertical lines over the sternum that are accentuated with the medial movement of both arms

Hands and Forearms

▶ To improve hyperpigmented macules (age spots)
▶ To improve superficial wrinkling
▶ To improve rough texture

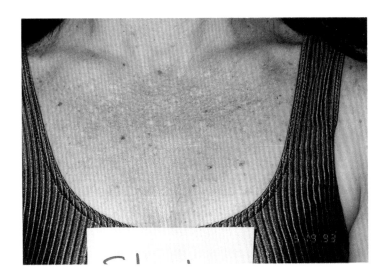

Figure 4-5

Hypopigmented acne scarring on the chest. Surrounding erythema and hyperpigmentation secondary to chronic photodamage are visible.

I have found sunburn freckles to be extremely unresponsive to bleachers and to peeling, including papillary dermal peeling. I have given up trying to treat these lesions with peels or bleaching agents. These lesions sometimes improve with cautious cryotherapy with liquid nitrogen. At this time, the newer pigment lasers may be the best therapy.

I have also found acne scarring on the back to be fairly unresponsive to TCA peeling. Although other physicians have claimed good success in this area, I have yet to see good before and after photographs documenting these results (especially 3 months postpeel when the edema has disappeared). In addition, I have seen back peels cause scarring. Therefore, I recommend that patients with acne scarring on the back not undergo peeling unless they are willing to accept small amounts of improvement on the order of 10% to 20%.

Certainly, any level peel will improve the roughened texture of actinically damaged skin. For that matter, an aggressive regimen of retinoic acid, AHAs, or both can do the same over a longer period of time. Dr. Cherie Ditre showed significant thickening of the dermis in forearm skin of patients treated with 25% AHA cream for 6 months.

If the patient truly has superficial wrinkling on the hands or arms due to atrophy of the epidermis and papillary dermis, it is possible that repetitive epidermal peels may help them. Dr. Paul Collins showed that repetitive intraepidermal peels can induce collagen formation in the papillary dermis. Similarly, clinical improvement is seen in these lines with repeated light peels. However, these lines do not disappear completely, and deeper lines fail to improve at all.

The hyperpigmented lesions on the dorsal hands and forearm will respond to peels to varying degrees (Fig. 4-6). Careful examination of these lesions with 3× magnification shows that a significant number of these age spots, or "liver spots," are actually slightly elevated seborrheic keratoses, which do not respond well to

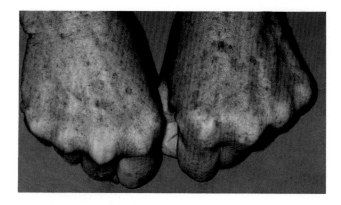

Figure 4-6
The dorsal right hand shows a moderate reduction of hyperpigmented lesions 6 weeks after one 30% TCA peel (level 2).

intraepidermal peeling. Attempting to peel off the entire epidermis with any agent other than resorcinol or salicylic acid is fraught with danger since dermal peels in this area often scar.

I have yet to see excellent results from dermal peeling of the hands. They all seem to have an abnormal textural change. Similarly, in medical meetings, I have not seen honest before and after photographs showing an effective dermal peel of the hand without some abnormal sequelae.

Please do not misinterpret this information and conclude that chemical peeling of the hands or other nonfacial area is ineffective. It is a useful superficial adjunct to other modalities for improving texture, color, and fine lines. If both you and the patient are willing to undergo several intraepidermal peels, the results can be quite gratifying.

SAFETY PRECAUTIONS

1. Always check the label on the bottle of any chemical you are applying to a patient's skin. Accidental application of the wrong acid can create serious problems.
2. Never pass an open container of acid (or an applicator wet with acid) over the patient's face. It is possible to accidentally drip acid onto the skin.
3. Never perform a peel with the patient lying completely flat. Always elevate the patient's head at least 45 degrees. Failure to elevate the head increases the chances of acid collecting around the eye.
4. Always have water nearby to flush the eyes in case acid gets into them.
5. Watch for tears with all peels. A tear running down the cheek onto the neck can create an area of peeling on the neck.
6. If you change brands of peeling agents (or change pharmacists making the solutions), always be sure you know whether the preparation is made by the same weight/volume measurement. With glycolic acid, it is important to note whether the pH of the new solution is the same as the pH of the previous one.
7. Before peels, always ask patients whether
   a. they recently had a facial waxing
   b. they recently used a facial depilatory
   c. they recently had electrolysis
   d. they recently had head or neck surgery
   e. they have taken isotretinoin (13-cis-retinoic acid; Accutane) within the past 1 to 2 years
   f. they are currently using retinoic acid (Retin A) or alpha hydroxy acids
   If the answer to any of these questions is yes, the patients may react more strongly to a peel.
8. Any peel patients with a history of herpes simplex should use oral acyclovir (even with light peels).
9. All patients undergoing any type of treatment for photodamage must use a broad-spectrum sunscreen *daily*.

Manual of Chemical Peels: Superficial and Medium Depth, by Mark G. Rubin. J.B. Lippincott Company, Philadelphia, © 1995.

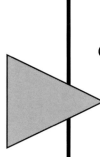

CHAPTER 5

PATIENT INFORMATION

Photographs ▶ *Checklists* ▶ *Consent Forms* ▶ *Instructions*

This chapter contains the written materials your office staff will need to assist you in performing peels in your office. It has examples of checklists, patient information sheets about different peels, patient instruction sheets for caring for peels, and consent forms.

▷ Photographs

If you do any type of cosmetic procedure, good-quality photographs are a necessity. No one, including the patient, really remembers what he or she used to look like. It is amazing how often a patient will point out a "new" nevus or telangiectasia that turns out to have been present on the before photographs.

Any patient undergoing any type of peel (or even just using a take-home regimen of alpha hydroxy acids and retinoic acid) should have at least three photos taken—one direct frontal shot and three-quarters oblique views of each side of the face (Fig. 5-1). Slide film rather than print film should be used for the most true-to-life color reproduction. (Ektachrome gives a truer tone to pigmented lesions than Kodachrome; Fig. 5-2). Most patients, however, find it easier to look at a print than a slide, so taking both slides and prints is advisable. Obviously, every effort should be made to standardize photographs by using the same camera, film, F-stop, light source, and background in all cases (Fig. 5-3).

If the patient is undergoing multiple peels or is having the home care regimen changed, he or she should be photographed before every procedure to document ongoing changes. The expense of a photograph is minimal, and it can be of tremendous value later. Inserting a self-adhering plastic sleeve inside the patient's chart to hold the photos is easy and makes them readily available.

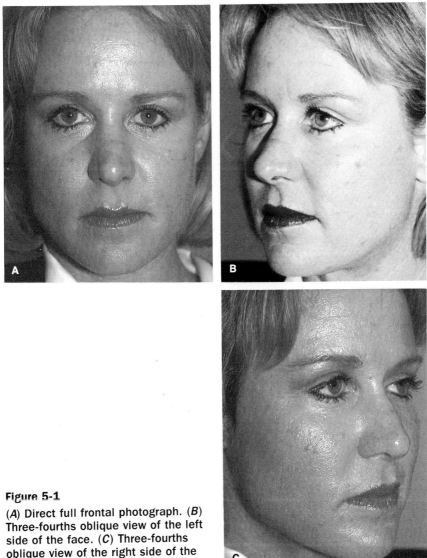

Figure 5-1

(A) Direct full frontal photograph. (B) Three-fourths oblique view of the left side of the face. (C) Three-fourths oblique view of the right side of the face.

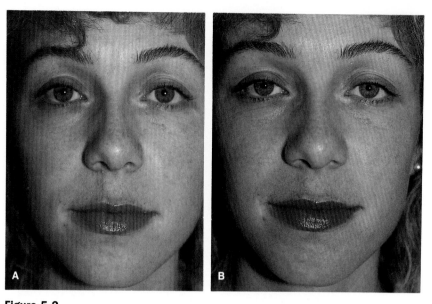

Figure 5-2

(*A*) Full frontal photograph of a woman taken with Kodak Ektachrome 100 ASA film. (*B*) Full frontal photograph of the same woman taken with Kodak Kodachrome 100 ASA film. The Kodachrome film develops with a yellower tone to the skin and decreased clarity of hyperpigmented areas.

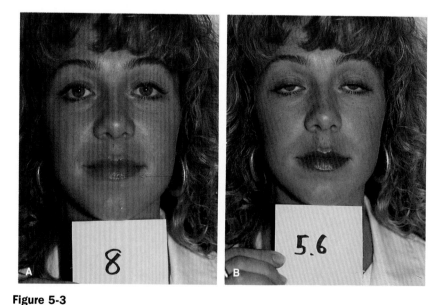

Figure 5-3

(*A*) Photograph taken with Ektachrome 100 ASA at F-stop 8. (*B*) Photograph taken with Ektachrome 100 ASA at F-stop 5.6. The lower F-stop produces a lighter skin tone, giving an artificial "freshening effect."

▷ Checklists

Contained in this chapter are some samples of checklists for physicians and assistants to use when performing medium depth peels to be sure that nothing has been overlooked. You can use these as they are or adapt them in any way you wish.

▷ Consent Forms

Any patient undergoing a procedure that has any risk of a complication should sign a consent form. Close adherence to this rule can be very helpful. If you are ever involved in a lawsuit and you do not have a signed informed consent, you're in serious trouble. Therefore, it makes sense to give patients the following:

- ► Written information about the type of peel they will undergo
- ► An instruction sheet detailing how to care for the peel
- ► A consent form describing the risks and benefits of the procedure

I have included several consent forms for both light and medium depth peels. Because medium depth peels are associated with more complications and more downtime, consent forms for them should be more in-depth. In particular, any consent form for medium depth or deep peels should include at least the following points:

- ► What benefits the patient can expect from the procedure
- ► How unpleasant the procedure and postoperative period will be
- ► How much downtime is normally required for healing (ie, how much work the patient should be prepared to miss)
- ► How the patient will look during healing
- ► What the risks of the procedure are

▷ Instructions

Having patient education materials and appropriate instructions for wound care can save you and your office staff a great deal of time. In addition, it will decrease the number of phone calls to your office from peeling patients. **An educated patient is always a better patient.**

The peel information sheets can also be mailed or given to prospective patients before their consultation to allow them to understand the procedures better. We also use brochures and instructional videotapes to educate patients before their consultation.

KEY POINT CHECKLIST

1. Did the patient block out enough time for their healing?

2. Does the patient have an underlying disorder that may slow down healing so he or she needs an additional 1 to 3 days to heal (ie, diabetes, kidney disease, heavy smoking)?

3. Is the patient's life peaceful or stressful at the time of the peel? (Moving, getting fired or divorced, and other stresses create a poor healing environment.)

4. Does the patient have the appropriate ointments and antibiotics or are prescriptions needed? (Most patients prefer to have all of their materials on hand *before* the peel so they don't have to wait in a pharmacy after the peel.)

5. Is the patient allergic to any antibiotics?

6. Does the patient has a history of herpes? (In which case, a prescription for acyclovir [Zovirax] is needed.)

7. Have all of the patient's questions been answered? Is he or she ready to undergo the peel or a bit hesitant? (A patient who is uncertain about being peeled on the day of the peel should not be treated; it's asking for trouble.)

8. Is the peel consent form signed?

9. Do you have good photographs (three views in both prints and slides)?

10. Has the patient been primed with retinoic acid, alpha hydroxy acids (AHAs), or hydroquinone as planned?

11. Have you determined what strength of peel you are planning to perform and what areas you may want to peel differently (eg, Jessner's solution, trichloroacetic acid, AHA)?

12. Have you determined what the postpeel care will be (eg, retinoic acid, bleaches, cortisone)?

13. Does the patient have any cuts, insect bites, or inflamed acne lesions that will interfere with the peel?

14. Has the patient had any neck or facial surgery in the past 3 months?

15. Have you given the patient *another* care instruction sheet?

PREPEEL CHECKLIST

Patient name: _____   Today's date: _____

Scheduled date of peel: _____   Photos taken: Prints_____ Slides_____

Is patient using:

    Retinoic acid?   0.025%   0.05%   0.1%   Cream   Gel

    Hydroquinone 4%?   Yes   No

    Alpha hydroxy acid and hydroquinone or alpha hydroxy
acid and kojic acid?   Yes   No

Has patient ever taken Accutane?   Yes   No

    If yes, when? _____

    Dosage: _____

Is patient allergic to any antibiotics?   Yes   No

    If yes, which ones? _____

Does patient have history of herpes?   Yes   No

Has patient had recent surgery?   Yes   No

    If yes, what type and when? _____

Prescriptions given to patient today:

    Hytone ointment   _____

    Cetaphil/hytone lotion   _____

    Antibiotic:

        Type:_____

        Dosage:_____

        Acyclovir:_____ (if needed)

Consent given?_____Care instructions given?_____

Patient reminders for medium depth peel

    1. Patient advised to take two aspirins 30 minutes before peel?   _____

    2. Patient advised to come to office without any makeup?   _____

    3. Does patient have a quiet week at the time of peel?   _____

    4. Patient reminded to wear open-necked, comfortable clothing?   ____

    5. Patient reminded to bring a hat?   _____

DAY-OF-PEEL CHECKLIST

Patient name: _____   Today's date: _____

Did the patient pick up all prescriptions and over-the-counter products?	Yes	No
Has the patient signed the consent form?	Yes	No
Have photographs been taken?	Yes	No
Does the patient have a quiet week coming up?	Yes	No
Has the patient had any recent illness or surgery?	Yes	No

If yes, what?_____

Has the patient taken aspirin today?	Yes	No
Does the patient have any unanswered questions about the procedure?	Yes	No

If yes, what?_____

Patient's skin cleaned with:

   10% Glycolic acid solution   _____

   Alcohol   _____

   Acetone   _____

   Hibiclens   _____

Care instructions gone over with the patient?	Yes	No

Remind patient:

   Sleep on back   _____

   Shower with caution   _____

   Minimize facial expressions   _____

   No exercising   _____

   No picking   _____

   Avoid sunlight   _____

   Call office if they have any questions   _____

Schedule peel recheck:

   Date and time: _____

SETTING UP THE PATIENT FOR A PEEL

The following is a checklist for the office assistant. It includes items to remember so the patient will be prepared when the physician enters the room to perform the peel.

1. Let the patient know he or she will be in the room for about 1 hour. Ask if he or she needs to use the restroom at this time.

2. Make sure the patient is wearing loose clothing around the neck.

3. If the patient is wearing contact lenses, ask whether he or she wishes to remove them, since the eyes may tear.

4. Check whether the patient has taken the prepeel aspirin yet. If not, ask him or her to do so at this time (if not aspirin-sensitive).

5. If the patient has worn makeup to the office, have her wash it off.

6. Check whether the peel consent form has been signed and whether the patient has any questions or concerns.

7. Clean the patient's face according to the physician's instructions.

8. Reassure the patient that everyone is usually nervous at this time.

9. Ask whether the patient has picked up all the required prescriptions and over-the-counter products.

10. Take photographs if none are in the chart from the prepeel check-up. (If you do not see them, they may not have been developed properly.)

SETTING UP THE ROOM

As with any office procedure, it is best to be prepared with all items the physician or patient might need. The following is a list of items most frequently needed during a peel.

Required

Small glass beaker or shot glass (to hold the peeling agent)
Well-marked bottles of peeling agent
Neutralizing solutions or lotions for each acid
Gloves (nonsterile gloves are fine for these procedures)
2×2 cotton gauze sponge
Cotton-tipped applicators (nonsterile)
Small sable hair or synthetic fan brush
Cleansers
    Alcohol
    Acetone
    Freon
    Hibiclens
    10% Glycolic acid solution
Kleenex
Blanket or towel (in case the patient becomes chilled during the procedure)
Hair band (to hold the patient's hair off the face)
Camera (in case the doctor wants photographs taken during the procedure)
Fans (either handheld or electric)
Examination table or chair set at a 45-degree angle
Ointment, emollients, or low-strength cortisone cream (to be applied immediately after the peel)
Container of water (to flush the eyes in case of accidental acid spill or drip)

Optional

Ice packs (to apply to the neck and chest of patients feeling flushed)
Glass of ice water for patient
Water-soaked compresses (to apply to peeled areas if they sting persistently)

PEEL CAUTIONS

A skin peel is a complex procedure with certain inherent risks. If you follow your doctor's advice and directions, the risk of complications in this procedure is small. Anything that you do against doctor's advice increases the chances of your having complications.

You will be well informed as to what you can and cannot do during peeling. It will be your responsibility to follow this advice since you will be caring for your skin at home.

There are certain conditions that may require postponement of your peel. These include

▶ inflamed acne lesions
▶ open cuts or scratches on your face
▶ active cold sores on lips or face
▶ any facial surgery within 3 months, including a facelift or eyelid surgery

In addition, if you are under severe physical or mental stress, it is not a good time for a peel. It is important that you can devote all of your energies to your peel and are not distracted by other physical or mental needs.

It is extremely important that you do not pick, scratch, pull, or rub your skin during your peel. If you do, you may damage the underlying new skin and cause scarring or changes in your pigmentation.

If, despite these warnings, you pick or rub your skin, you may ruin your peel. The doctor may elect not to perform any further peels on you if there is doubt that you will follow instructions exactly.

Please realize that these warnings are for your protection. The motto in this office is **if you are not sure if you should do something or don't understand the directions, call the office before you do anything!** We never think that any of your questions are foolish or silly.

INFORMED CONSENT FOR ALPHA HYDROXY ACID PEELS

I understand that I am going to have a light glycolic acid (alpha hydroxy acid) peel. I understand that this is a superficial type of peel that normally creates, at most, only 1 or 2 days of mild redness with occasional areas of flaking skin.

I understand that on rare occasions this peel can penetrate deeper in certain areas, causing a crusted scab to form. I understand that if this area is not treated appropriately it could become infected and possibly lead to the formation of a scar. It is my responsibility to contact the doctor's office if any crusted areas form or if my skin does not look and feel completely normal within 3 or 4 days after my peel.

I am undergoing this peel in an effort to improve my skin texture and color. I understand I may achieve some improvement in my fine wrinkles as well, but no guarantee has been made to me regarding my level of improvement from this peel. The doctor has explained to me that I may need several of these peels to achieve my best results.

_____

Patient Signature   Date

_____

Witness Signature   Date

INSTRUCTIONS FOR CARE DURING ALPHA HYDROXY ACID PEELS

You have just had a light glycolic acid peel. Because of the superficial nature of this peel, you should not expect to really "peel." Most patients who undergo this therapy have only a little redness for 12 to 24 hours. Occasionally, they may have very slight flaking in a few localized areas for 1 or 2 days. In rare instances, an area of crusting may develop. If this occurs, apply an antibiotic ointment, like Polysporin or Bacitracin, to the area and notify our office if it fails to improve within 24 hours.

During the entire time of your healing, you should apply a bland moisturizer to your skin as often as needed. Do not apply any medications or glycolic acid products during this time or your skin will become irritated.

Do not expect to see much reaction to this peel. Most patients look normal the day after a glycolic acid peel. The maximum benefit of this procedure is not really apparent until about 2 or 3 weeks after the peel.

INFORMED CONSENT FOR JESSNER'S PEELS

I understand that I am going to have a Jessner's peel performed on my _____. I understand that this is a superficial type of peel that will make my skin feel dry, flake, and peel for anywhere from 2 to 7 days, depending on the depth of my peel. I understand that during the time I am healing I will look a bit red in my peeled areas and it may be difficult for me to cover it up with makeup.

I understand that on very rare occasions this peel can penetrate deeper in certain areas, causing a crusted scab to form. I understand that if this area is not treated appropriately it could become infected and possibly lead to the formation of a scar. It is my responsibility to contact the doctor's office if I develop any crusted area.

I am undergoing this peel as part of a program to improve the texture and color of my skin. The doctor has explained to me that I may need several peels to achieve my best results, and no guarantee has been made to me about the degree of improvement I can expect to see.

_____   _____
Patient Signature   Date

_____   _____
Witness Signature   Date

INSTRUCTIONS FOR CARE DURING JESSNER'S PEELS

Jessner's peeling is a chemical treatment designed to remove superficial layers of skin. It is used to help dry out active acne, to reduce shallow wrinkling and scarring, and to lighten hyperpigmented, dark patches on the skin.

Before the solution is applied, your skin is cleaned with alcohol and then glycolic acid. It would be helpful if you would not wear any facial makeup to the office on the day of your treatment.

The solution is applied to your skin with gauze, cotton applicators, or a small brush. Because the solution is a combination of mild acids, some stinging usually occurs during application. After the solution is applied, your face may have white areas called frosting. This shows that the solution is working and usually fades within 15 to 30 minutes. Your face may appear slightly redder than usual for some time after the treatment.

In most cases, peeling usually occurs between the second and fifth days after a treatment. Your skin will probably become very dry, and some small cracks may develop. The doctor recommends a nondrying cleanser, such as Dove, Neutrogena, or Cetaphil, and proper moisturizer, such as Complex 15, Lubriderm, Nutraderm, or DML. You may apply makeup as usual. In general, the peeled area will appear mildly or moderately sunburned.

As you continue with light peel treatments, they will be spaced at 2- to 4-week intervals. The number of treatments required for any given problem varies with each person and is determined by the patient and the doctor. The number of coats of solution varies with skin type. It is impossible to know in advance how much peeling will occur, but if you note the relative amount of peeling that occurs after each session, future peels can be adjusted to suit your needs. There is no limit to the number of peels a person can receive as long as improvement continues.

You may continue to wear makeup after light peel treatment. You should also continue using oral medicines, but topical medications such as retinoic acid (Retin A) and glycolic acid should not be applied for several days after your peel.

Your skin is a living organ, made up of millions of cells. Everyday, thousands of cells die, fall off, and are replaced by new cells from below. This is a slow and haphazard process that does not allow your skin to shed dark spots, sun damage, or a dull, lifeless complexion.

The purpose of a facial peel is to cause the even, controlled shedding of several layers of damaged cells, so you are left with a new fresh layer of skin, with a more even texture and color. This process is similar to a snake shedding its skin.

Many types of facial peels have been performed in this country during the past 20 to 30 years. The most common peel, called a *chemical peel,* uses the chemical *phenol* as its peeling agent. This potentially toxic chemical creates a deep peel and usually caused the skin to become permanently lighter in color and often rather blotchy. In addition, the texture of the skin often becomes waxy and masklike.

The facial peel performed in my office does not use phenol. The main ingredient is trichloroacetic acid (TCA). This creates a peel that offers less risk of scarring and pigmentation changes than the phenol chemical peel. Because the peel I perform is not as deep as a phenol peel, it is not as effective in improving deep wrinkles, but it can make marked improvements in blotchy pigmentation, freckling, sun damage, fine wrinkles, and some types of acne scars. When you have healed after a TCA peel, you should have skin that is your own natural color and texture.

The peel is an outpatient procedure performed in my office. It consists of the application of one or several layers of medication to your skin to create a controlled chemical burn. There is normally a few minutes of stinging and burning after the medication is applied. This usually stops within 2 or 3 minutes, and there is no more discomfort during the rest of the time you are peeling, although most people experience itching during the healing process. During the next several days, your skin turns darker, feels tight, then cracks and peels off, leaving you with a new fresh layer of skin. There are no scabs, bleeding, or bandages.

During healing, you should have no pain. Most people look strange during peeling, but if you don't mind your appearance, you are able to go out and even go to work. However, you will not be able be in the sun or do anything that would cause you to perspire heavily.

The average peel takes 5 or 6 days to complete. Deeper peels, for heavily sun-damaged and wrinkled skin, may take 8 or 10 days. There are specific medicated creams you will need to use during peeling. You will be supplied all of this information on another sheet.

Most patients require more than one peel to achieve their best improvement. For most skin types, two peels are needed to give the best results, but some skin problems, such as excessive pigmentation from pregnancy or birth control pills, may require multiple peels for maximum improvement. Everyone's skin is different, so each person's peel program is tailored to his or her individual needs. When I examine your skin I will tell you what I believe needs to be done for your skin to accomplish what you desire.

INFORMED CONSENT FOR TRICHLOROACETIC ACID FACIAL PEELS

A skin peel is not a "cure all" treatment, but for appropriate conditions, it can give you marked improvement. It is important that you have a thorough understanding of what the peel can and can't do for your particular condition. I, _____, give my consent for Dr. _____ to perform a skin peel on my face or other area of my body _____ to treat the following conditions:

_____.

_____ The peel program was explained to me in detail. I have seen photographs of patients taken before, during, and after the peel treatment.

_____ Dr. _____ has explained to me what benefits I can realistically expect to see from my peel program, including _____

_____.

I understand that this is a program of treatments and that I may need several peels to achieve my best results.

_____ I understand that the degree of improvement I can expect to see depends on many variables and therefore cannot be guaranteed. Additionally, I understand that strict adherence to the doctor's instructions is necessary to ensure my best results.

_____ I understand that Dr. _____ has the right to discontinue my treatment at any stage if he or she thinks that I am not following instructions, or if he or she believes that no further improvement is possible.

_____ I understand that the skin peel is an outpatient procedure done in the office, that consists of the application of medications to the skin. I understand that I can expect to have 1 to 2 minutes of stinging or burning sensations immediately after the medication has been applied, but this will stop.

_____ I understand that during healing from my peel, my skin will look darker and shiny and that I may be unable to work. My particular peel and its relationship to my ability to work have been discussed with me by Dr. _____ .

_____ I consent to have my photographs taken before, during, and after my treatment. These may be used for educating future patients and in possible publications and promotions. My name will not be used.

_____ Although complications are rare, they occur. Prompt recognition and treatment of any complication is necessary to decrease its potential danger. It is extremely important that I follow doctor's instructions exactly and that I notify the office if I have any of the following complications:

▶ Skin infections—usually appearing as a red tender area, often with a scab
▶ Cold sore on my lips or face
▶ Allergic reaction to any medications I am using in conjunction with the peel
▶ Appearance of thick scars or keloids in the areas of my peel
▶ Prolonged sensitivity to the wind and sun
▶ Persistent areas of increased or decreased pigmentation

_____   _____
Patient Signature   Date

_____   _____
Witness Signature   Date

INSTRUCTIONS FOR CARE DURING TRICHLOROACETIC ACID FACIAL PEELS

Make sure you have your prescription daily lotion, 3% hydrogen peroxide, and Hytone ointment or other moisturizer. In addition, you will need 5 to 7 days' worth of antibiotics to take during your peel.

Use the recommended soap to wash your face gently for 20 to 30 seconds twice a day. Lather the soap in your hands and gently pat it onto your face, then splash lukewarm water onto your face to rinse. Dry your face by patting it gently with a clean towel. If you have been instructed to use 3% hydrogen peroxide (which reduces the chance of getting an infection), use it diluted (mixed half and half with clean water) after washing your face twice a day. Gently dab it onto your face with cotton balls or gauze. It will bubble and may turn white. If hydrogen peroxide is too irritating and stings, you can dilute it even more with clean water.

After washing and patting your face dry, apply the daily lotion in the morning and at night. After the daily lotion has soaked in, apply Hytone ointment as instructed. Apply the Hytone ointment gently; don't rub it in hard. You should use the ointment as often as necessary to keep your skin from getting dry and cracked. We'd rather you be too greasy than not greasy enough. Don't let your skin dry out, it will pull on the new tissue underneath and may cause red, irritated areas. You can apply your ointment 10 times a day if you want! This will reduce the tightness and will make you more comfortable. Don't worry if all the ointment doesn't come off when you wash your face; it won't harm you to leave some on. You may develop occasional whiteheads because of all the ointment on your skin. This is normal, do not be alarmed since they will resolve over time. Also, be aware that some mild itching and burning is normal at this time.

Be sure and minimize facial expressions during your peel. Excessive facial movements will cause the skin to crack prematurely. This is not a good time to see a funny movie, visit your dentist, or eat a hero sandwich.

Don't pick or rub your skin at all. If you must wash your hair, wash it with your head tilted backward in the shower or in the sink. Do not wet your face in the shower, too much water will cause you to peel prematurely and will leave you with red, sore areas that may lead to scarring or need to be treated again. If large pieces of peeling skin are hanging from your face, they may be cut off carefully with a pair of blunt-nosed scissors. Do not sit in a sauna or jacuzzi or do strenuous exercise at this time. Sweating will make your face sting and it will cause you to peel too soon.

Do not expose your face to sunlight at all during healing. If you have to do some exercise, you may go out for a walk in the early morning or late evening when the sun is barely out.

During peeling, think of your dark old skin (which is peeling off) as a bandage that protects the fresh new skin underneath. The longer you can keep this natural bandage in place, the better will be the results of your peel.

You may have some swelling during the first 2 or 3 days after your peel, particularly if it is a medium or deep peel. In extreme cases, your eyes may swell almost closed during the first two mornings. This is a normal response and will resolve on its own, but sleeping with an extra pillow to elevate your head may help to decrease swelling in the meantime. **Do not apply ice packs or cold compresses to your face to decrease the swelling.** The moisture from these may cause the skin to peel prematurely.

It is important that you try to sleep on your back so you don't rub your peeling skin against the pillow. This could create an area of prematurely peeled skin.

After the peel, sunscreen must be used to protect the skin from the rays of the sun. You need to use it even if you are wearing a hat, since the reflected rays may also cause damage. Please request sunscreen samples if they were not given to you before your peel.

Makeup may be used 1 or 2 days after peeling is complete. We will recommend when you can wear it.

If you have unexpected irritation or possible infection, call the office immediately! **Do not wait until your next appointment.** This is especially important if you think you may be developing a cold sore on your lip.

If you are experiencing a lot of itching, be sure you use plenty of Hytone ointment. You may also try using your daily lotion four or five times a day. (Refrigerating your lotion will make it feel more soothing.)

Summary

1. Continue to wash your face twice a day with soap and lukewarm water. Don't try to wash off very bit of the Hytone ointment.

2. Use your daily lotion throughout peeling, in the morning and evening.

3. Keep your face very moist with Hytone ointment or another moisturizer that we recommend.

4. Do not pick or rub your skin.

5. Do not go out in the sun at all while peeling, even for 5 minutes!

6. Do not use the cleaning or moisturizer routines as excuses to speed up peeling of your skin through excessive rubbing; it will only increase your risk of complications.

7. Don't be alarmed if you feel flushed or warm when you bend over. This is a temporary condition that resolves after the peel has healed completely.

Products to Apply to the Skin During Healing

Monday   AM:

PM:

Tuesday   AM:

PM:

Wednesday   AM:

PM:

Thursday   AM:

PM:

Friday   AM:

PM:

Saturday   AM:

PM:

Sunday   AM:

PM:

Additional instructions:

Manual of Chemical Peels: Superficial and Medium Depth, by Mark G. Rubin.
J.B. Lippincott Company, Philadelphia, © 1995.

CHAPTER **6**

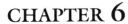

JESSNER'S PEELS

Jessner's Solution ▶ *Performing the Peel* ▶
Complications

JESSNER'S SOLUTION

Formula

▶ Salicylic acid, 14 g
▶ Resorcinol, 14 g
▶ Lactic acid (85%), 14 g
▶ Ethanol to make 100 mL

Stability

▶ Retains strength for up to 2 years if container is opened only 5 minutes a month
▶ Light- and air-sensitive; may develop a salmon-colored tint on exposure to light and air so it should be stored in a dark amber bottle with a tight cap

Physical Characteristics

▶ Light amber solution that darkens with age and exposure to air and light
▶ Distinct medicinal smell

▽

JESSNER'S PEELS

Pros

+ It is very difficult to overpeel a patient and inadvertently create too deep a wound.
+ Jessner's peel creates a good deal of exfoliation (which some patients like to see).

Cons

− Because the formula contains three active ingredients, there is a greater chance of manufacturing variations.
− There is possible toxicity from resorcinol.
− There is possible toxicity from salicylic acid.
− For such a superficial peel, it creates a significant amount of stinging and burning and is more uncomfortable than 10% trichloroacetic acid (TCA).
− Jessner's peel creates a good deal of exfoliation (which some patients don't like to see).

△

▷ Jessner's Solution
James Dolezal, MD

Jessner's solution is a preparation used as for light peels alone or in preparation for a TCA peel. It contains resorcinol USP, salicylic acid USP, and lactic acid USP, 14% each in ethanol USP. It is a clear, pale to medium yellow-pink solution with an alcoholic odor. Fresh resorcinol should be used because resorcinol turns dark with exposure to light and air. Salicylic acid is light-sensitive. Trace amounts of ferric iron turn salicylic acid red.

Because salicylic acid, resorcinol, and lactic acid are solids, computation is weight in volume (W/V). Lactic acid USP is a liquid that contains, by weight, 85% lactic acid, an alpha hydroxy acid, in water. When the USP preparation is used, the actual concentration of lactic acid is 15% less than the labeled percentage of the USP preparation. A source of error would be to compensate for this by using 18% lactic acid USP, to provide the equivalent of 14% of lactic acid crystals. This would be an error because the formula calls for 14% lactic acid USP. If the lactic acid, with a density of 1.2, is measured by volume instead of weight, a preparation 20% stronger than the standard will result. Incorporating both of these errors at once would result in a preparation that is over 40% stronger in lactic acid than the standard. Lactic acid absorbs water in moist air, and use of old lactic acid can result in a subpotent preparation.

The vehicle, ethanol USP, is considered by the federal government to be of beverage quality and therefore subject to the taxes normally levied on 190- to 200-proof alcoholic products. Because of its high cost, few pharmacies stock or use this grade of ethanol, opting instead to use inexpensive denatured alcohol. Denaturing alcohol is a process whereby various substances are added that render the alcohol unfit for beverage purposes. Most denaturants are chosen so that they cannot be removed in ordinary distilling processes. Denaturing agents include methyl isobutyl ketone, pyronate, gasoline, acetaldol, and kerosene. Unauthorized recovery of pure ethanol is discouraged by keeping secret the actual denaturing agents in any given preparation. If denatured alcohol is used in preparing Jessner's solution, it is not possible to predict what interactions might occur.

▷ Performing the Peel

Skin Preparation

As with all peels, the results will be best if the skin is primed before the peel. The goals of skin preparation for all patients set to undergo peeling are as follows:

1. Epidermal turnover should be enhanced.
2. The stratum corneum should be thinned.
3. Oil and debris should be removed.

As previously described, skin preparation should consist of the use of retinoic acid, alpha hydroxy acid, or a combination of both. In addition, a bleaching agent should also be used if you are treating the patient for a dyschromia. Remember, this is a light peel, so there is no need to aggressively prime the skin and induce erythema and scaling. If the skin is primed too aggressively, you may inadvertently create a deeper peel than you desire.

Cleaning

Thoroughly clean the skin to remove makeup, oil, and debris. This can be done with alcohol, acetone, freon, chlorhexidine, or other cleansers. Since this is meant to be a superficial type of peel, there is no need to do an aggressive scrub to clean the skin. The goal is to degrease the skin, not to strip off any remaining stratum corneum.

Application

In a standard Jessner's peel, the solution is applied to the skin with a sable-hair brush. The solution can also be applied with cotton-tipped applicators, 2×2 gauze squares, cotton balls, or many other applicators. Whatever applicator is used, the goal is to apply a uniform layer of acid to the entire area of skin surface to be peeled. I have found that a synthetic fiber brush works as well as a sable-hair brush. I have left a synthetic fiber brush completely submerged in Jessner's solution for 3 months, and the fibers remain intact. However, there is a concern about the use of a nondisposable brush to perform these peels. Patients may have superficial abrasions, scabs, or pustules on the face, any of which could contaminate the applicator brush. Unfortunately, the brushes do not stand up well to repeated sterilization. Therefore, it seems prudent either to dispose of the brush after each peel or to use another type of disposable applicator.

Rubbing the Jessner's solution into the skin with a 2×2 gauze square enhances the penetration of the solution (Fig. 6-1). Therefore, in patients with

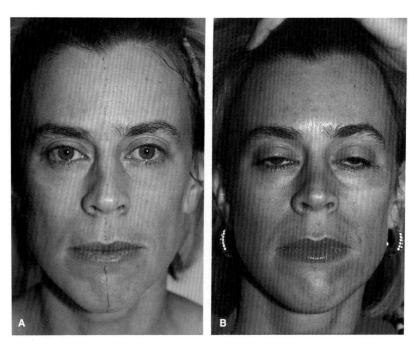

Figure 6-1

(*A*) A woman 10 minutes after two coats of Jessner's solution were applied with a sable brush on the patient's right side and rubbed into the skin with a 2×2 gauze on the left side. (*B*) The same patient 2 days later. The areas of erythema and hyperpigmentation are more pronounced on the patient's left side in the infraorbital and chin area (the side to which the acid was applied with a gauze sponge). This is evidence of the increased depth of wounding achieved by rubbing the acid into the skin.

thick, sebaceous skin (who are more resistant to the penetration of an acid), applying the solution by aggressively rubbing it into the skin with a 2×2 gauze gives a deeper, more uniform peel. On the other hand, in patients with thin, sensitive skin, applying the solution with a softer applicator, like a paintbrush or cotton-tipped applicator, is a safer approach and one that is more comfortable to the patient.

End Point of the Peel

As the depth of a Jessner's peel increases, clinically apparent visual changes occur on the skin surface that correspond to the depths. The first response of the skin to a very superficial Jessner's peel is faint erythema. Associated with this may be a light, powdery-looking whitening on the skin surface. This is not a frost but presumably is the precipitation on the skin of one of the chemicals in the solution. This whitening can be wiped off with your finger or with water on a cotton ball (Fig. 6-2). It is important to differentiate this whitening from a true frost due to tissue coagulation. This level of peel (level I) is very superficial and will create only 1 or 2 days of mild flaking or sometimes even no flaking at all.

As the Jessner's solution penetrates deeper with the application of additional coats, erythema becomes more pronounced, often turning bright red rather than pink. At this time, some fine, pinpoint areas of true white frost usually become visible (Fig. 6-3). Normally, patients feel a mild to moderate amount of burning and stinging with this level of peel. This stinging persists to some degree for 15 to 30 minutes, although on occasion some patients may feel persistent mild stinging or sensitivity for several hours.

During the next 1 to 3 days, skin subjected to this level of Jessner's peel (level 2) usually develops a persistent mild red-brown coloration, occasionally with the streaking previously mentioned. For 2 or 3 days, the skin feels like a layer of

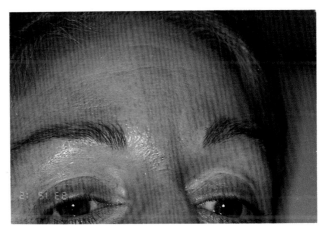

Figure 6-2

White precipitant on the skin associated with a level 1 Jessner's peel. Note the area in the mid-forehead where the precipitant was easily wiped off with a damp cotton ball. It is important to differentiate this whitening from a true frost, which cannot be wiped off (see Fig. 6-4).

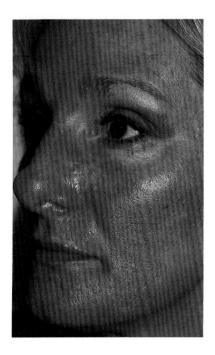

Figure 6-3

Level 2 Jessner's peel showing pronounced erythema and scattered small areas of true white frost (most pronounced along the temple and the side of the chin).

plastic film has been applied, and then it exfoliates for an additional 2 to 4 days. Normally, the skin appears windburned, with moderate flaking, but actual peeling is rare.

The next depth (level 3) of Jessner's peeling shows prominent erythema with a significant number of pinpoint areas of frosting, creating a notable whitish look to much of the surface of the skin (Fig. 6-4). Most patients feel a moderate amount of stinging with this level of a peel.

During the healing phase, skin undergoing a level 3 Jessner's peel looks and feels similar to that with a level 2 Jessner's peel. However, the exfoliation may last as long as 8 to 10 days. Some significant actual peeling may also be seen with this peel rather than just dry, flaking skin. Crusting and weeping are not seen with even a level 3 Jessner's peel, however, since it is an intraepidermal peel.

The depth of a Jessner's peel is related to the preparation of the skin prior to peeling, the thickness of the stratum corneum, the sensitivity of the skin, the number of coats of solution that are applied, and the method of application. In most cases, it takes one coat of Jessner's solution to get a level 1 peel. It may take two or three coats to achieve a level 2 peel, and three or four coats to achieve a level 3 peel. Obviously, there is some variation in these numbers based on the skin type being peeled and other factors previously mentioned, but it is fairly unusual to have one coat of Jessner solution create a level 2 or 3 peel. It is far more common that it may take multiple coats of solution to achieve a level 1 peel. I have seen some patients take six coats of Jessner's solution to achieve a level 1 peel.

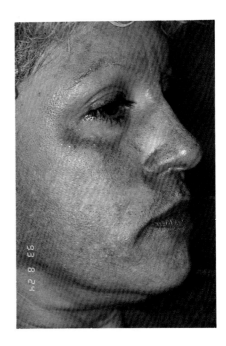

Figure 6-4
Level 3 Jessner's peel showing marked erythema and a
moderate amount of white frost.

It takes 4 to 6 minutes for the full skin reaction to occur after applying the
Jessner's solution. Any additional coats of the solution should not be applied until
you have waited that long to evaluate the skin and to determine how deep a peel
you have already created.

Postpeel Care

Because most patients feel that their skin is tight and masklike, frequent use of
creamy emollients is helpful. The peeling skin may be a little sensitive, so staying
with bland, fragrance-free moisturizers like Neutrogena, DML, Complex 15, and
Theraplex is best. Certainly, petrolatum and vegetable shortening are alternative
emollients, but they are cosmetically unacceptable to most people undergoing a
light peel and they preclude the use of any makeup. If the patient has persistent
sensitivity or stinging, a mild topical steroid cream or ointment can be used two
or three times a day to calm the skin.

During the healing phase of the peel, patients can attempt to wear makeup
(after applying a moisturizer) but definitely cannot use scrubs, masks, astringents,
toners, or retinoic acid or alpha hydroxy acid products. They can resume use of
any of these products 48 hours after the peel has healed.

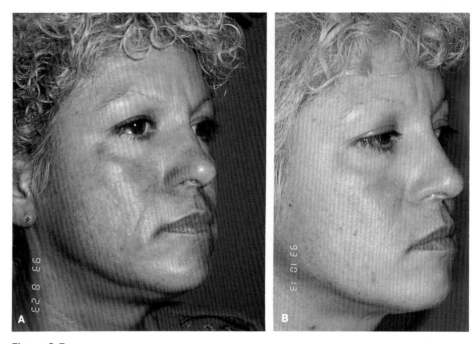

Figure 6-5

(*A*) A woman with persistent epidermal melasma despite the use of alpha hydroxy acids, retinoic acid, and 4% hydroquinone. (*B*) The same woman 7 weeks after a level 3 Jessner's peel. Marked improvement in hyperpigmentation is seen.

Why Use Jessner's Solution?

The Jessner's peel has been popular to varying degrees for many years. Recently, there has been a upswing of interest in it. Although a Jessner's peel is seldom more effective than a similar depth peel with TCA, it has certain benefits that should be matched to the appropriate patients:

1. They are very superficial and *rarely* go deeper than you expect. So a Jessner's peel is a safe choice for patients with thin, sensitive skin.
2. They create a fairly uniform depth peel (unlike AHAs).
3. They create a good deal of exfoliation. This is helpful in treating dyschromias, when you are trying to decrease the number of melanin-containing keratinocytes (Fig. 6-5).
4. Since the concentrations of resorcinol in Jessner's solution is low, there is less risk of toxicity than with a regular-strength resorcinol peel.

Caution

As a general rule, Jessner's peels create flaking or peeling. This is a peel for someone who wants to "peel." Even a light Jessner's peel makes the skin shiny and tight for a few days, followed by several days of exfoliation. In addition, the resorcinol component of the peel often creates mild erythema, usually a red-brown color, which can persist throughout the entire duration of peeling. The erythema and discoloration associated with this peel have a tendency to be streaky, making it more unsightly and more difficult to cover with makeup.

▷ Complications

Because a Jessner's peel is a superficial peel, complications are rare. As stated earlier, it is difficult for a peel to accidentally go too deep with Jessner's solution. I have seen only one case of a Jessner's peel that penetrated into the dermis, and that was a thin-skinned woman who had 12 coats of this solution applied to her neck at one sitting by an esthetician.

The most common complaints associated with Jessner's peels are not really complications. They are persistent irritation or stinging, streaky erythema, and slow peeling. True complications are allergic reactions, systemic toxicity from resorcinol or salicylic acid, infection, and persistent erythema.

Allergic Reactions

Of the three chemicals in Jessner's solution, resorcinol had been stated to have the greatest tendency to cause allergic reactions. Most physicians advocate patch tests (in the postauricular area) with any resorcinol-containing compound several days before the actual peel. I have performed more than 1000 Jessner's peels and have never seen an allergic reaction, implying that the rate of allergic reactions is less than 0.1%. Other physicians who do a great deal of peeling with resorcinol agree with my experience.

Toxicity

A more in-depth discussion of toxicity is found in Chapter 2. However, a brief overview of toxicity follows. Of the three chemicals found in Jessner's solution, resorcinol and salicylic acid have the potential to create systemic toxicity. The true potential for toxicity is based on the amount of the chemical absorbed into the skin. Because most of the cleaning and priming of the skin done before the peel is designed to enhance the penetration of Jessner's solution into the skin, the only real variable is the surface area treated and the number of coats of solution that are applied.

A review of the literature on Jessner's peels shows repeated references to the need to limit the size of the area treated to prevent resorcinol toxicity. In reality, salicylic acid toxicity (salicylism) is the limiting factor. Even when peeling the face, neck, and chest with several coats of Jessner's solution, the safety profile is quite good. However, salicylicism has been seen with simultaneous Jessner's peeling of the face, chest, arms, and lower legs.

Infection

The chances of an intraepidermal wound becoming infected are remote. Therefore, an uncomplicated Jessner's peel should not become infected. If a patient excessively rubs his or her peeling skin or accidentally traumatizes it, however, the wound may be extended into the dermis, increasing the potential for infection.

If a wound becomes infected, treatment should include local wound care in conjunction with topical and systemic antibiotics. (For more detailed information, see Chapter 10.)

Persistent Erythema

In a small number of patients, some degree of erythema is present in areas for several weeks after the peel. This mild erythema from superficial peels, which fluctuates in intensity during the day, is not cause for concern. It is not the same as the deeply red or violaceous persistent erythema that can complicate medium depth peels, leading to hypertrophic scarring.

The degree of erythema changes throughout the day. It is usually at its best in the morning when the patient first arises, and it worsens with face washing, exercise, and consumption of hot beverages, alcohol, and spicy foods. Basically, anything that enhances blood flow to the face worsens the erythema.

Erythema is a rare complication of Jessner's peels and is always self-limited. Usually, the patient's skin feels normal with no increased sensitivity or tightness. Low-strength topical corticosteroid creams (desonide [Desowen], hydrocortisone butyrate [Locoid]) or bland emollients are the only therapy needed other than daily use of sunscreens.

Manual of Chemical Peels: Superficial and Medium Depth, by Mark G. Rubin.
J.B. Lippincott Company, Philadelphia, © 1995.

CHAPTER 7

GLYCOLIC ACID PEELS

Neutralization ▶ *Glycolic Acid Strength and pH* ▶
Performing the Peel ▶ *Complications*

GLYCOLIC ACID

Formula

▶ Glycolic acid/hydroxy ethanoic acid crystals at 100% (reagent grade, not cosmetic grade)
▶ Highest cosmetic grade is a 70% solution, Glypure, made by DuPont
▶ Solutions are made using water or a combination of water, alcohol, and propylene glycol

Stability

▶ Not light-sensitive, so it does not need to be stored in a dark bottle
▶ Very stable (more than 2 years)
▶ Deliquescent (absorbs moisture from the air), so it must be kept tightly capped

Physical Characteristics

▶ Clear solution; can be made into a gel with addition of a gelling agent
▶ Gel may look a little yellow or cloudy

▽

Glycolic acid peels

Pros

+ Even very superficial glycolic acid peels may be able to achieve significant effects.
+ Peels are well tolerated by patients.
+ Glycolic acid produces no systemic toxicity.

Cons

− There is tremendous variability from patient to patient in reactivity and efficacy.
− Glycolic acid does not always create actual peeling of the skin (not always necessary for results).
− It has to be neutralized
− It has a tendency to penetrate unevenly.

△

Alpha hydroxy acids (AHAs) are a group of organic acids, some of which are derived from fruits, hence their name—fruit acids. Despite the fact that glycolic acid can be found in sugar cane, the glycolic acid used in your practice is not derived from processing sugar cane. It is created in a laboratory from chemical reagents, that is, bubbling carbon monoxide through formaldehyde. (So much for the concept of a "safe" plant extract.) Below is a list of acids and their natural sources:

> *Glycolic*—sugar cane
> *Lactic*—sour milk
> *Citric*—citrus fruit
> *Malic*—apples
> *Tartaric*—grapes

These products are often used in 8% to 15% concentrations as part of a daily regimen of skin care. However, they can also be used as peeling agents.

When we speak of AHA peels, we are usually speaking about glycolic acid. Although there are peeling solutions made up of pure lactic acid or of mixtures of other AHAs (eg, lactic, citric, and malic), most AHA peels are done with glycolic acid.

Glycolic acid as a peeling agent, rather than a daily skin care product, usually is in a concentration of 30% or greater. Glycolic acid peels using concentrations of 30% to 50% are often performed by estheticians (cosmetologists) or nurses, whereas peels using 50% to 70% glycolic acid are generally performed by physicians. As with all other nonphenol peeling agents, the higher the concentration of the acid, the more aggressive its action and the deeper the peel; that is, a 70% glycolic acid peel is a more aggressive peel than a 30% glycolic acid peel performed on the same patient.

AHA peels are useful in the treatment of many conditions in addition to photodamage. However, here I will focus on their use in the treatment of the clinical signs of photodamage, including rough, textured skin; dyschromias, and fine wrinkling. At this time, AHA peels are probably the most commonly performed peels in the world, certainly in the United States. This is due to the following factors:

1. They are systemically safe, nontoxic acids.
2. They are usually very superficial peels, and hence have few complications.
3. The lay press has written extensively about them, creating a great deal of consumer interest and demand.

▷ Neutralization

Glycolic acid peels (all AHA peels) need to be neutralized to terminate their action when they have achieved the desired depth of wound. If you leave them on the skin, unneutralized, they may penetrate too deeply and "overpeel" the patient.

Neutralization can be done using any product with an alkaline pH (a base neutralizes an acid) or by flushing the area with water and diluting the acid. The use of an alkaline neutralizer provides fairly rapid resolution of any stinging or burning from the glycolic acid peel, whereas rinsing the face with water fails to provide the same rapid resolution of the stinging. In addition, by actually neutralizing the acid and terminating its effect, there is no chance that the peel will continue to penetrate. Washing the face with water may not remove all of the glycolic acid on the skin (particularly if it is in a gel form), inadvertently leading to areas of deeper peeling.

I use an assortment of neutralizing agents, including products called "peel neutralizer lotions" from Dermatologic Cosmetic Labs and Veritas. In addition, I use 10% to 15% solutions of sodium bicarbonate (NeoStrata, Pharmagen). The products are equally effective, but each has it pros and cons.

Sodium Bicarbonate Solution

In the process of neutralizing the acid, sodium bicarbonate solution creates carbon dioxide, seen as bubbling or fizzing on the surface of the skin (Fig. 7-1). If

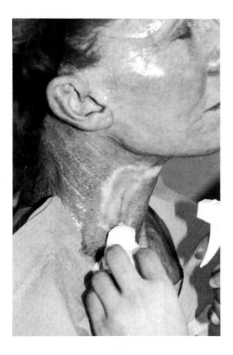

Figure 7-1

A 70% glycolic acid peel on the neck being neutralized with a 10% sodium bicarbonate solution. The white bubbling signals that neutralization is occurring in the area in which the bicarbonate has been applied.

you continue to apply the liquid solution until the fizzing stops, you can be assured you have neutralized all the acid. The drawback to sodium bicarbonate solution is that it must be applied in copious amounts to the entire peeled area. The solution ends up dripping all over and making quite a mess. In addition, the neutralization of glycolic acid with sodium bicarbonate is an exothermic reaction that generates heat, making the patient's face more erythematous and potentially inducing a deeper wound.

Other Neutralizing Agents

The neutralizing lotions are much more cosmetically elegant to use since they can be applied to the face with gauze squares or large cotton-tipped applicators and they do not drip onto the neck and chest. The drawback is that they produce no clinically visible sign of neutralization, like fizzing, to indicate whether the product is working or when all of the acid has been neutralized.

For these reasons, I often apply sodium bicarbonate solution with cotton-tipped applicators to areas in which the peel must be terminated immediately and then apply a neutralizing lotion to the rest of the face. Once either type of neutralizer has been applied, I have the patient go to the sink and wash this mixture from his or her face with a large amount of cool water.

▷ Glycolic Acid Strength and pH

Histologic studies performed on mini pigs by Larry Moy at UCLA showed that 70% free glycolic acid left on the skin for 15 minutes created a dermal wound as deep as 40% trichloroacetic acid (TCA). This means 70% glycolic acid can create a papillary dermal wound if it is left on the skin unneutralized for too long.

Because the depth of a glycolic acid peel is time-dependent, if you neutralize a 70% glycolic acid peel rapidly, it can give you the same depth of peel and the same results as a 50% glycolic acid peel left on the skin for a longer time. Therefore, it is far safer to start by using 50% glycolic acid left on the skin longer than to start with 70% glycolic acid that may have to be removed or neutralized rapidly to prevent overpeeling.

Several companies make glycolic acid peels. In addition to various strengths from 30% to 70%, a choice of free acid solutions or partially neutralized solutions is available. Part of the confusion about AHA peels is that no one has demonstrated in a scientific study whether peels with free acid are more effective than those with partially neutralized solution.

The solutions containing free acid have significantly lower pH values than those containing partially neutralized acid. As an example, M.D. Formulations Physician Exfoliating Solution 70% glycolic acid (containing about 48% free acid) has a pH of 2.75%. NeoStrata Skin Rejuvenation System 70% glycolic solution contains all free acid and has a pH of 0.6. NeoStrata 50% solution (containing about the same amount of free glycolic acid as M.D. Formulations 70%) has a pH of 1.2. The lower-pH products create more burning, stinging, irritation, and erythema than their counterparts with higher pH values. Clinically, this means most patients cannot tolerate the acids left on the skin for as long as they could solutions with a higher pH. Also, there is more of a tendency for solutions with very low pH to penetrate unevenly, causing areas of accidental deeper peeling.

Because there is no scientific documentation of which solution is best, you will have to make your own decision. The routine that I currently follow may not be considered the most effective 2 years from now, but at this time it seems to work the best for me.

CAUTION

▶ Glycolic acid 70% can create an uneven peel.
▶ Glycolic acid 70% can create a dermal wound.
▶ Glycolic acid 70% can create scarring (I have seen several cases).

▷ Performing the Peel

Skin Preparation

As with all peeling agents, patients preparing to undergo a glycolic acid peel should have their skin primed for at least 2 weeks before the peel. Your choice of products includes retinoic acid, AHAs, and bleachers, depending on the patient's skin type.

Cleaning

Because these peels are generally intended to be superficial, the cleaning regimen is a degreasing routine, not an "epidermabrasion."

Application

When performing glycolic acid peels, it is important to remember that you must neutralize this peel to terminate its action. Therefore, before you begin an AHA peel, **always be sure you have your neutralizing agent close by**. If you forget to have your neutralizer in the room, the peel may become too deep while you try to find it.

Glycolic acid peeling solutions come in solutions and gels. I prefer using a gel because it has less tendency to drip after it has been applied to the face.

The actual application of glycolic acid to the face should be performed rapidly. Since you will be attempting to create a uniform peel, it is important to apply the acid to the entire face for a similar amount of time. If it takes 2 minutes for you to apply the acid to the entire face, some areas will have been exposed to the acid for 2 full minutes and other areas will have only 5 seconds of exposure. This is obviously going to create an uneven peel. Therefore, your goal should be to apply the acid to the entire face within 15 to 20 seconds.

As a safety precaution, it is best to start applying the glycolic acid in an area that is least reactive or sensitive. The forehead usually can safely tolerate 15 to 30 seconds more exposure to the acid than the cheeks or chin. By starting the application on the forehead and rapidly applying the glycolic acid to the rest of the face, you increase the chances of a uniform peel. Neutralizing the peel by area in the same order that you applied it also helps keep the acid exposure time fairly constant over the entire face.

The acid can be applied with a brush, cotton-tipped applicator, or gauze squares (Fig. 7-2). Fan brushes have become the most popular applicator, but they are not easy to sterilize and should be disposed of after each use. If you use a cotton-tipped applicator, a large swab or scopette works well, since either has to be dipped in the solution only one time to hold enough solution to peel the entire

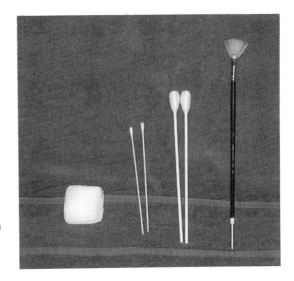

Figure 7-2

Several types of applicators commonly used in performing a glycolic acid peel (*left to right*): 2×2 gauze, cotton-tipped applicators, scopettes, fan brush.

face. (A lot of time is wasted redipping the smaller cotton-tipped applicator in the acid several times.)

The depth of the glycolic peel does not appear to be related to the volume of the acid applied (unlike TCA). You can overlap areas without concern of accidentally inducing a deeper peel. However, some physicians believe that massaging or rubbing an area with the applicator enhances the penetration of the acid.

Once the acid has been applied to the entire face, your job is to constantly examine the face, looking for "hot spots," or areas of erythema or epidermolysis that need to be neutralized. If there are only one or two of these areas, they can be neutralized and the rest of the peel left to continue penetrating. Once there are three or more of the hot spots, I neutralize the entire peel. Not all patients develop hot spots. Some experience a more uniform erythema. However, it is helpful to have the patient tell you if any areas of their skin are burning more than others. These are areas to watch closely, because increased discomfort usually is associated with an area of deeper penetration.

During the time the acid is in place on the skin, most patients feel some tingling, itching, or mild stinging. This can be alleviated with the use of a hand-held or power fan. Once the acid has been neutralized, any discomfort should stop fairly rapidly.

What strength glycolic acid should I use? Because many of the patients who come to my office have already had 30% to 50% glycolic acid peels performed by an esthetician without achieving the results they desire, I usually use 70% glycolic acid in an effort to produce a more aggressive peel. Also, since I have many years of experience with glycolic acid, I am not worried about using the strongest glycolic acid peel and accidentally overpeeling a patient.

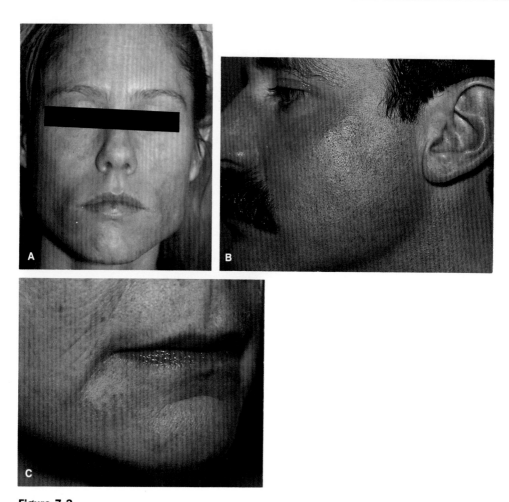

Figure 7-3

Clinical signs associated with glycolic acid peels of increasing depth. (All peels were performed with 70% free glycolic acid.) (*A*) Patchy areas of pink coloration 2 minutes after application. (*B*) Pronounced erythema at 2½ minutes. (*C*) Area of white epidermolysis below the oral commissure at 3½ minutes. (*D*) Erythema and vesiculation at 2½ minutes. (*E*) Erythema and patchy areas of true white frost on the cheeks at 3 minutes.

If you are just starting with glycolic acid peels, the safest strength to start with is 30%, but this is a very weak peel and may not produce any significant improvement. Therefore, I suggest starting with 50% glycolic acid. The higher-pH M.D. Formulations 70% solution (which is really 48% free acid) is well tolerated by most patients. If the patient tolerates this strength peel for 7 to 10 minutes with only mild erythema, I would use 70% free glycolic acid for his or her next peel.

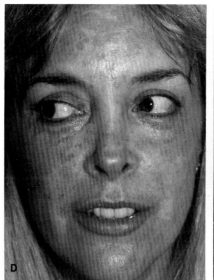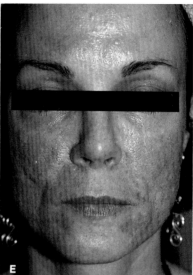

Figure 7-3 (Continued)

How long do I leave the acid on? There is no easily definable definite end point to AHA peeling. The stages of glycolic peels in increasing order of depth of peel are pink, red, epidermolysis and vesiculation, frosting (Fig. 7-3). Erythema corresponds to some level of intraepidermal wounding, with red being deeper than pink. Epidermolysis shows as a gray-white color in areas in which the epidermis has separated from the dermis and has become hydrated (similar to the appearance of your fingertips after being submerged in water for a prolonged time). Vesiculation is due to epidermolysis and signifies the same depth of wound. True frosting seems to be an indicator of dermal injury, but there are no scientific studies to support this conclusion.

If your goal with AHA peeling is to create a smoother skin surface with improved clarity or translucency of the skin, you really need only to thin the stratum corneum with a very light AHA peel. Light AHA peels have an end point of mild erythema.

If you are trying to remove some hyperpigmented areas from the skin, you may actually want to create necrosis in the superficial epidermis to destroy some of the melanin-containing epidermal cells. In this situation, the end point of the peel is scattered areas of punctuate epidermolysis of the skin, signifying epidermal necrosis. These areas heal with crusting over 4 to 7 days (Fig. 7-4). However, if a peel is intended to improve postinflammatory hyperpigmentation, this level of glycolic acid peel is deep enough to create new inflammation and possibly new areas of hyperpigmentation.

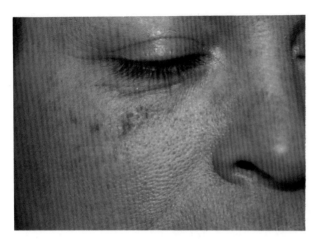

Figure 7-4
Area of mild crusting of the right infraorbital area 48 hours after a 70% glycolic acid peel that created an area of epidermolysis below the right eye.

If your goal is to get significant improvement in wrinkling, you usually need to create significant epidermal necrosis with concomitant dermal inflammation. This level of AHA peel shows an end point of large areas of white epidermolysis. These peels take 5 to 7 days to heal and are crusted during that time (Fig. 7-5). This depth peel also has increased risk of complications since it is a more aggressive peel.

Some patients can tolerate 70% free acid for 8 minutes with no erythema and other patients develop vesiculation in 2 minutes. The most important rule in glycolic acid peeling is **never leave the room during the peel!** You must continually watch the patient's skin for clinical signs of wounding from the peel. Don't be obsessed with timing the peel. Be aware of what the skin looks like, and terminate the peel when you observe the end point you desire, no matter how short or long the acid has been on the skin.

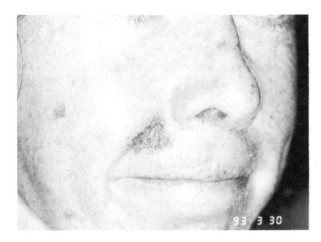

Figure 7-5
Large crusted area in the upper nasolabial fold 72 hours after a 70% glycolic acid peel that created marked epidermolysis in this area.

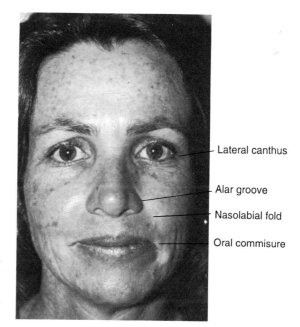

Lateral canthus

Alar groove

Nasolabial fold

Oral commissure

Figure 7-6
Areas of the face that show greater reactivity to glycolic acid peeling: alar groove, nasolabial fold, lateral canthus, oral commissure, and the area just inferior to the oral commissure.

Areas of the skin that have a thinner stratum corneum, underlying xerosis, or dermatitis absorb the acid faster than the rest of the skin. This is commonly seen in the alar groove, the nasolabial fold, lateral canthus, oral commissures, and the area just inferior to them on the chin (Fig. 7-6). Therefore, if one area on the face shows erythema or epidermolysis before the rest of the face, you should neutralize that area only and allow the AHA on the rest of the face to continue to penetrate.

Postpeel Care

If the patient has any irritation, erythema, or superficial crusting after the peel, he or she should not apply any of the daily AHA products or retinoic acid. If significant inflammation is present, a mild topical steroid cream (Hytone, Desowen, Aclovate) can be applied twice daily to speed resolution. If there are areas of crusting, the patient should be treated with a topical antibacterial ointment (Polysporin, Bactroban) three or four times a day and examined every 1 to 2 days until healed to ensure that no infection develops.

If the patient's skin looks fairly normal after the peel but feels a bit tight or sensitive, using a bland emollient two to four times daily for 1 or 2 days is all that is needed. As soon as the skin looks and feels normal again, the patient can restart his or her normal maintenance regimen of AHAs.

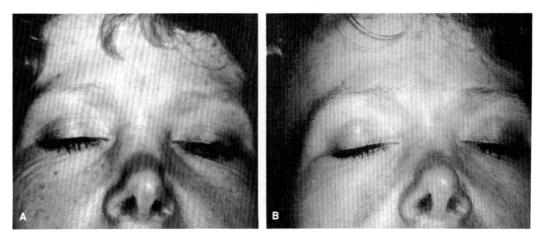

Figure 7-7
(*A*) A woman with fine wrinkles below the eyes. (*B*) The same woman 2 months after a
2-minute 70% free glycolic acid peel and 10% glycolic acid gel applied twice a day.

What areas of the body can be peeled with glycolic acid?   It appears that any area of
sun damage may be improved with glycolic acid peeling. Commonly, the face,
neck, and chest are peeled in many patients. The dorsal hands are also often
treated. Glycolic acid peels can help mottled hyperpigmentation and very fine
wrinkling on the neck, chest, and hands. However, significant wrinkling and
prominent age spots have been resistant to therapy in my experience. Remember
to avoid creating a dermal wound when peeling nonfacial areas, because these
wounds are prone to create scarring.

How many glycolic peels should I do?   Unfortunately, no one knows the answer to
this question. Some patients respond better than others to AHA peeling. I have
found that if the patient fails to improve after two AHA peels, he or she usually
will not improve with additional AHA peels and needs to be treated with a more
aggressive peeling agent. If the patient does improve after two AHA peels, he or
she should continue to be peeled until no evidence of additional improvement
with each peel is seen. (Obviously, photographic documentation of the patient's
improvement is necessary to make these determinations; Figs. 7-7 and 7-8.)

How often should glycolic acid peels be performed?   Again, no one knows the answer. Because it takes at least several weeks for dermal inflammation to resolve
after a peel, it makes sense to wait that long between peels to see what effects have
occurred on collagen or glycosaminoglycan deposition.

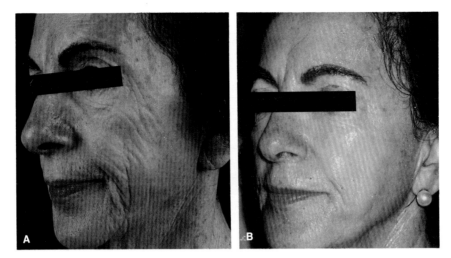

Figure 7-8

(*A*) A woman with level 3 photodamage before any therapy. (*B*) The same woman after 22 70% glycolic acid peels during a 2-year period. Each of these peels created patchy areas of epidermolysis. (Courtesy of Dr. Romulo Mene)

How painful are glycolic acid peels?   Glycolic acid peels generally sting or are mildly irritating, not painful. There is never a need to sedate a patient undergoing this type of peel. However, 70% free glycolic acid with a pH of 0.6 is quite irritating to some patients and can be moderately uncomfortable for a few minutes. The use of a handheld fan normally keeps these patients comfortable.

Are certain patients at risk for an accidentally deeper penetrating glycolic acid peel?   Absolutely yes! Patients with histories of sensitive skin, particularly those who have trouble tolerating a daily 8% to 10% glycolic acid cream, react strongly to even a low-dose, 50% glycolic acid peel. In addition, patients who have been primed aggressively with AHAs, retinoic acid, or salicylic acid absorb the peel more rapidly. This tendency is also seen in patients who use facial masks or exfoliating scrubs. Finally, any area of the skin that has been recently wounded with harsh chemicals (hair dyes, depilatories, permanents, straighteners, or waxes) will have deeper penetration of the acid.

> ## KEY POINTS FOR GLYCOLIC ACID PEELS
>
> **1.** Glycolic acid can create dermal wounds. Don't ever tell a patient it is a risk-free peel.
> **2.** Glycolic acid peels usually need to be repeated several times for their best effect.
> **3.** Some patients get significant effects from glycolic acid peels, other patients do not.
> **4.** AHA peels are variable in terms of their results. Therefore, it is best to try to undersell the results when discussing them with a potential peel candidate.
> **5.** Glycolic acid peels always need to be neutralized to terminate their action.
> **6.** They can create significant inflammation in some patients and can induce postinflammatory hyperpigmentation.

▷ Complications

The complications seen with glycolic acid peels are the same as those seen with other peels, such as TCA (see Chapter 10). However, most complications are related to the depth of the peel. If you perform only superficial glycolic acid peels, you should have few complications and none should be serious. Potential complications from glycolic acid peeling include the following:

Herpes labialis: Since a glycolic acid peel is an acid burn on the face, a herpes infection may be triggered. Prophylactic acyclovir (Zovirax) in appropriate patients is justified.

Persistent erythema or sun sensitivity: This is extremely rare and is self-limited.

Inadvertent overpeeling in areas: Superficial crusting similar to a rug burn can be created in areas of epidermolysis. It should be treated with topical antibiotics as for any other crusted wound. The patient may be unhappy to develop crusting from a peel if he or she was expecting a so-called lunchtime peel with no downtime.

Postinflammatory hyperpigmentation: This is not common with superficial glycolic acid peels since they rarely create significant inflammation, which is the precursor to this type of hyperpigmentation.

Infection: This is a rare complication unless the patient is accidentally overpeeled and the wound is cared for inappropriately.

Scarring: Scarring is extremely uncommon with glycolic acid peels. It is due to either dermal wounding from the peel or the development of an infection that is not treated appropriately.

Manual of Chemical Peels: Superficial and Medium Depth, by Mark G. Rubin.
J.B. Lippincott Company, Philadelphia, © 1995.

CHAPTER **8**

SALICYLIC ACID PEELS (NONFACIAL)

Salicylic Acid Paste ▶ *Performing the Peel*

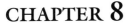

SALICYLIC ACID

Formula

▶ Salicylic acid powder USP, 50%
▶ Methyl salicylate, 16 drops
▶ Aquaphor, 112 g

▽

Salicylic acid peels

Pros

+ Salicylic acid peels are technically easy to perform.
+ They have a low incidence of significant complications.
+ It is difficult for the peel to penetrate too deeply.
+ They are effective for the treatment of hyperpigmented age spots on the hands and arms.

Cons

− It is unpleasant for patient to have an arm wrapped for 48 hours.
− They have a long healing time (as with all peels of the arms or hands).
− Salicylism is fairly common.

△

▷ Salicyclic Acid Paste

Salicylic acid is used at 14% strength in Jessner's solution and at 2% strength as a skin cleanser. A third form is used for peeling, that of a 50% salicylic acid paste to peel the arms and hands. Salicylic acid peeling of the arms and hands has been in the US literature since the early 1980s but has never become popular. Part of the reason may be the unwillingness of the physician and patients in this country to accept the use of pastes in chemical peeling. (There is also a poor level of acceptance for resorcinol paste peels in the United States.) The safety and efficacy of salicylic acid arm peels was demonstrated by Swinehart in 1991. He reported on 92 patients who underwent peels with salicylic acid paste with good results and no significant complications.

Peels of the arms and hands can be the most frustrating peels to attempt. Repetitive superficial peels using Jessner's solution, glycolic acid, or trichloroacetic acid (TCA) 10% to 20% are not particularly efficacious. More aggressive peeling with higher-strength TCA can give much better cosmetic results but carries with it a higher incidence of the development of hypopigmentation, textural changes, or obvious scarring. Indeed, the healed skin of most arms and hands that have undergone papillary dermal peels looks slightly abnormal. For this reason, many physicians tell patients that there is no acceptable therapy for photodamage of the arms and hands. Other physicians may elect to treat individual hyperpigmented lesions with cryotherapy, using liquid nitrogen. Cryotherapy is an excellent treatment option for age spots, but it is unpleasant and time-consuming when treating multiple areas. In addition, inadvertent overtreatment can create hypopigmented areas or scars.

The most common complaints among patients requesting peels of the arms and hands are

- age spots
- actinic keratoses
- fine wrinkling
- deep wrinkles and loss of elasticity

Salicylic acid paste peeling adequately addresses the first two or three of these complaints. (I don't think any peel can safely improve significant wrinkles and loss of elasticity on the hands or arms.)

▷ Performing the Peel

Skin Preparation

Mild forms of salicylism are common with this peel, so only one arm should be peeled at a time. As with all peels, the skin needs to be primed before the peel for a minimum of 2 weeks. Most patients easily tolerate retinoic acid on the arms, so they should have no problem using retinoic acid 0.05% to 0.1% cream every night. In patients with multiple hyperkeratotic lesions and rough skin, it is beneficial to also add a 10% to 15% glycolic acid gel in the morning. Because most of these patients have hyperpigmented lesions they want to improve, a hydroquinone or kojic acid product should also be used both before and after the peel. Most patients find it easiest to use a gel containing both an AHA and a bleaching agent in the morning and retinoic acid at night.

Cleaning

On the day of the peel, the skin on one arm or hand should be cleaned with an acetone scrub (using acetone on a 2×2 gauze, rubbed on the skin for 2 or 3 minutes). Any elevated hyperkeratotic lesions on the skin should be treated either with TCA 20% applied with a cotton tipped applicator or with light cryotherapy with liquid nitrogen using a brief 2- to 3-second freeze time. I have found that using liquid nitrogen is more effective than 20% TCA as a pretreatment of these lesions. **You must pretreat these areas to get the best results.**

Application

Once the skin has been cleaned and the thickened lesions pretreated, the next step is to protect the areas of skin you don't want to peel. This includes the volar

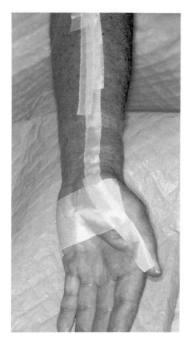

Figure 8-1

The volar forearm and wrist are protected by tape before the application of the salicylic acid paste.

forearm, lateral aspects of the fingers, and interdigital web spaces. This can be done by using petrolatum or tape as a protective barrier (Fig. 8-1). Cotton balls placed between the fingers protect the interdigital spaces. After these areas have been protected, the paste can be applied.

The paste is thick and is most easily applied with a wooden tongue depressor or spatula. It should be applied in a thick coat over the entire area to be peeled. In most patients, this includes the proximal fingers up to the proximal interphalangeal joint (Fig. 8-2). The next step is to occlude the peeled area with plastic wrap. This can be somewhat tricky to do on the hand. It may be helpful to poke four fingerholes in a sheet of plastic wrap and, after placing the fingers through the holes, to drape the wrap over the rest of the hand and arm and tape it in place (Fig. 8-3). Failure to adequately occlude the paste causes it to desiccate and to create a more uneven superficial peel. The final step is to wrap the entire treated area with a 4-inch-wide roll of gauze (Kling, Kerlix) to protect the peeled arm. This bandage is left in place for 48 hours.

Postpeel Care

During healing, the patient is instructed to drink at least eight glasses of water a day (to decrease the chance of salicylism) and to notify the office if experiencing nausea, disorientation, or tinnitus. The patient may experience some degree of

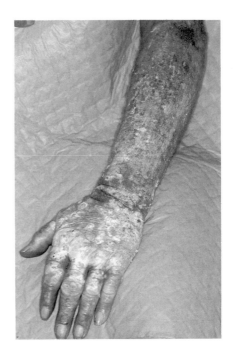

Figure 8-2

The appearance of the arm after the salicyclic acid paste has been applied. The paste is also applied up to the proximal interphalangeal joint.

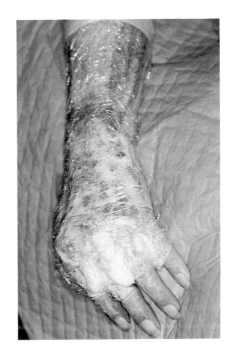

Figure 8-3

The appearance of the arm after the paste is covered with plastic wrap and taped in place. Cotton balls are placed in the interdigital area for protection of that skin.

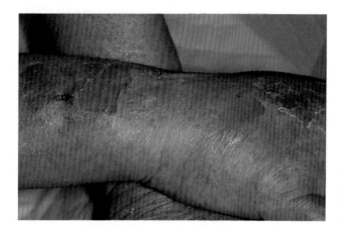

Figure 8-4
Seventy-two hours after the paste has been removed, the skin is edmatous and beginning to peel.

burning or stinging while the peel is taped in place, but it is rarely unpleasant enough for concern. It is imperative that you caution the patient not to take any aspirin for pain during this time.

After 48 hours, the patient returns to the office to have the bandage and plastic wrap removed. At this time, the skin usually appears macerated and edematous. Any identifiable remaining salicylic acid paste should be removed with gentle saline compresses. The entire peeled area is treated with a saline compress left on for 5 minutes, followed by application of a topical antibiotic ointment (Polysporin, Bacitracin) and a gauze wrap.

The patient is instructed to change the dressing daily by gently rinsing the arm in the shower (not letting the shower spray directly onto the arm), reapplying the antibiotic ointment, and rewrapping the area with gauze. The patient should be seen back in the office every 2 to 4 days to ensure he or she is healing well (Fig. 8-4). Any evidence of thicker crusting, erythema, or tenderness needs to be

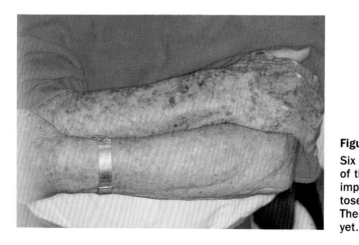

Figure 8-5
Six weeks after a salicyclic acid peel of the patient's left arm. Marked improvement is seen in actinic keratoses and lentigenes on the forearm. The right arm has not been treated yet.

treated with oral broad-spectrum antibiotics and stronger topical antibiotic ointments (Bactroban, Garamycin). **The skin in this area scars easily: do not let it get infected.**

Most hand and arm peels are healed in 10 to 16 days. At that time, the new skin is often somewhat mottled and may be quite red. It may take 4 to 6 weeks for the skin to really return to normal (Fig. 8-5). Once reepithelialization has occurred, the patient should begin using daily sunscreens and resume his or her maintenance program with retinoic acid, AHAs, and bleaches.

Once the patient is completely reepithelialized and there is no risk of infection, you can treat the other arm. On rare occasions, you may want to retreat an arm to achieve a better result. You can safely repeel an arm after waiting 2 to 3 months. If you repeel this area too soon, the peel is much more reactive and there is a greater chance of creating a deeper wound.

Manual of Chemical Peels: Superficial and Medium Depth, by Mark G. Rubin.
J.B. Lippincott Company, Philadelphia, © 1995.

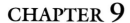

CHAPTER **9**

TRICHLOROACETIC ACID PEELS

Trichloroacetic Acid Solutions and Basic Pharmacy ▶ *Performing the Peel* ▶ *Nonfacial Peels With Trichloroacetic Acid* ▶ *Enhanced or Combination Peels*

TRICHLOROACETIC ACID

Formula

▶ Trichloroacetic acid (TCA) 30% (W/V) = TCA crystals USP, 30 g
▶ Added distilled water to total volume of 100 mL

Stability

▶ Not light-sensitive
▶ Refrigeration not needed
▶ Stable for at least 23 weeks in an opened container
▶ 20% to 100% TCA stored unopened in TCA-resistant clear plastic containers for 2 years has been found to be within 3% of the labeled strength

Physical Characteristics

▶ Colorless and clear
▶ Free of precipitate

TRICHLOROACETIC ACID PEELS

Pros

+ TCA causes no systemic toxicity.
+ It can be used to create superficial, medium, or deep peels.
+ It is inexpensive.
+ It is stable.
+ Peel depth correlates with intensity of skin frost.
+ There is no need to neutralize a TCA peel.

Cons

− Higher concentrations (over 40%) seem more apt to create scarring.

TCA has become the gold standard of chemical peeling agents (Fig. 9-1). It has been well studied; it is versatile in its ability to create peels of different depth; it is stable, inexpensive, and nontoxic.

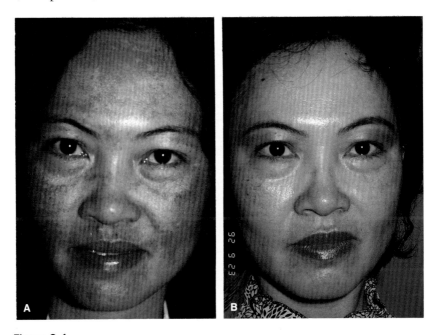

Figure 9-1

(*A*) An Asian woman with marked epidermal melasma despite the use of alpha hydroxy acids, retinoic acid, and hydroquinone. (*B*) The same patient 3 years after two level 2 TCA peels (using 35% TCA).

▷ Trichloracetic Acid Solutions and Basic Pharmacy
John Dolezal, MD

Because major manufacturers do not make a branded TCA solution in strengths appropriate for peels, physicians have relied on alternative sources. These include mixing by the physician, mixing by a local pharmacist, or purchasing a standardized preparation.

Arithmetic and measuring errors, use of old crystals, and contamination are potential sources of error for extemporaneously made preparations, whether compounded in a physician's office or local pharmacy. If, during preparation, the TCA crystals are left exposed to air before weighing, they absorb water and the final solution is weaker than intended.

TCA is no longer an official drug, having been deleted from the current USP (revision XXII). It last appeared as an official drug in a monograph in USP XXI. When used medically, TCA should be prepared from TCA crystals meeting the standards delineated in USP XXI. Old TCA crystals and industrial grades are not likely to meet these standards.

Simple arithmetical, weighing, or measuring errors are common. A bottle of TCA crystals can be partially used and remain on a pharmacy's shelf for years. Pure chemicals such as TCA crystals generally do not carry an expiration date. TCA is deliquescent, so a preparation made from old crystals with absorbed water would be subpotent. Hydrochloric acid is one of the decomposition products of TCA and could be present in old TCA crystals. TCA attacks cellulose, so TCA packaged in glass bottles with paper lined caps can react with the cellulose in the liner, resulting in contamination with unknown decomposition products.

If a physician uses a preparation that he or she makes (or that is made by a local pharmacist and always mixed in the same way), that preparation would be standard for that physician and he or she would be familiar with the action of that particular strength. However, if the physician is going to compare results with, or make alterations of, his or her technique based on the experience of another operator, a common basis for determining the actual strength of each preparation is essential.

In the dermatologic literature, four separate methods of mixing TCA solutions have been described, none of which provides the same absolute concentration of active material for any given strength. The variation of concentration between the weakest and strongest variation is nearly double.

The standard pharmaceutical method for computing the strength of a solution in which a solid is dissolved in a liquid is the *weight in volume (W/V) method*. By convention, such a solution is considered W/V even if not specifically indicated or stated. The standard methods of computing the strength of a solid incorporated in another solid is weight in weight (W/W), such as in ointments or creams. In the case of an ointment, a 1% concentration is considered to be W/W whether or not W/W is stated. When an author or physician claims he or she is using a 30% strength, the reader or listener should reasonably conclude that the preparation described contains 30 g of active material in each 100 mL of solution, 3 g/10 mL or 300 mg/mL.

However, authors have described several nonstandard methods of computing strengths of TCA preparations, all describing the solutions as a percentage. When one computes the actual W/V percentages, one author's "30%" may be considerably different from another's "30%." One such error is to describe a given percentage as being achieved by adding the same number of grams to 100 mL water; for example, claiming that 30% = 30 g with 100 mL water. Another error is to compute W/W the strength by adding a volume of water, considering it synonymous with a weight; for example, claiming 30% = 30 g with 70 mL (g) water. It is clear that 30 g dissolved in 100 mL water is not equivalent to 30 g dissolved in 70 mL water.

Another error is to describe the dilution of a saturated solution of TCA as a percentage; for example, claiming that 30 mL of a saturated solution mixed with 30 mL of water provides a 50% TCA solution. The actual W/V concentration actually obtained is not readily apparent. (It is actually about 74% W/V.) If used, such a solution should be labeled as follows:

Saturated solution trichloroacetic acid (USP XXI)	30 mL
Purified water	30 mL

or, alternately:

Saturated solution trichloracetic acid (USP XXI)	
Purified water	equal parts

Although these differences may seem trivial, inconsistencies in calculation have a significant effect on the resultant absolute concentration of the preparation. Because TCA is half again as dense as water, there is not a 1:1 relationship between TCA crystals or solutions and water.

By measuring the final volumes, the W/V concentration actually achieved using these different methods can be calculated and accurately compared.

Standard: 30 g TCA with enough water to make 100 mL solution, or 30% W/V

Aberration: 30 g TCA with 100 mL water makes 116 mL solution, which is the equivalent of 25.9% W/V

Aberration: 30 g TCA with 70 mL water makes 88 mL solution, the equivalent of 34.1% W/V

Aberration: 30 mL of saturated TCA solution (contains 43.23 g TCA) with 70 mL water makes 99 mL solution, or 43.67% W/V

In this example, the variation resulting in the strongest concentration is more than 65% stronger than the weakest.

TCA is not light-sensitive, nor does it require refrigeration. Dark brown bottles serve only to impede visualization of the contents. TCA solution should be clear, colorless, and free of precipitate or particles. They should be prepared from fresh crystals and stored in clear glass or TCA-resistant plastic bottles. Closures should use paper-free cap liners, such a TCA resistant-polyvinyl seal. TCA solutions should be prepared using the weight in volume (W/V) computations. Because compounding has been deemphasized in modern pharmacy training, if one is going to have a TCA preparation prepared by a local pharmacist, always specify weight in volume (W/V). Variation induced by use of old crystals and mathematical or computational errors can be avoided by obtaining TCA solutions in the desired concentrations from a supplier specializing in its preparation.

▷ Performing the Peel

Several peeling agents are commonly used to create superficial peels, but TCA is by far the most commonly used agent to create a medium depth peel.

Although TCA is occasionally used to create deep peels, it appears to induce a higher incidence of hypertrophic scarring than phenol. In addition, it can create hypopigmentation and a shiny skin surface, similar to that seen with phenol (Fig. 9-2). Therefore, deep peeling with TCA does not appear to have much advantage over phenol, with the exception of the lack of cardiotoxicity and the fact that TCA may create a bit less hypopigmentation than phenol.

The procedures for superficial, medium, or deep TCA peeling are similar, although the depth of the peel depends on many factors, including

- ▶ the patient's skin type
- ▶ how the skin was primed
- ▶ how the acid is applied
- ▶ how many layers of acid are applied
- ▶ how wet the applicator is with acid

The most important factor is the concentration of the TCA used. Keeping as many of the other variables as constant as possible allows the concentration of the acid to be the fundamental determinant of the peel depth. Therefore, the skin priming and cleansing should be the same for superficial and medium depth TCA peels.

Skin Preparation

The need for skin priming is as important for TCA peels as for other peels discussed in this manual. In particular, when performing medium depths peels

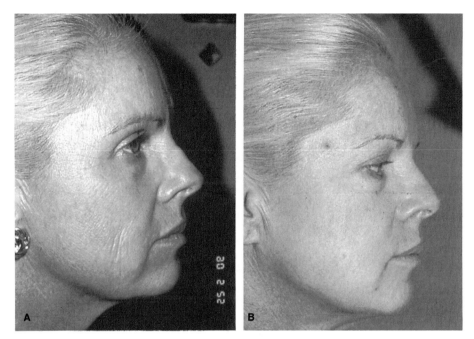

Figure 9-2
(*A*) A woman with level 2 sun damage with accordion pleat parallel smile lines on the cheek. (*B*) The same woman 6 weeks after her second level 3 TCA peel (using 40% TCA to the full face and 50% TCA applied directly to the mid-cheek wrinkles). There is an area of mild hypopigmentation on the cheek where 50% TCA was used.

with TCA, the benefits of priming (ie, increased speed of reepithelialization and decreased risk of postinflammatory hyperpigmentation) are even more important. Remember, the minimum amount of time needed to prime the skin for a peel is 2 weeks.

Cleaning

As with other peeling agents, the skin should be cleaned well before the peel. Once again, if the skin has been appropriately primed, and the stratum corneum is thin, there should be no need for an aggressive prepeel scrub. The degreasing and cleansing agent can be alcohol, acetone, Hibiclens, freon, or another agent.

Application

Once the skin has been cleaned, the patient should lie down on an examination table with the head elevated about 45 degrees. This angle keeps most patients more comfortable than lying flat on the back, and it seems to decrease the wave of heat associated with the hyperemic flush of a TCA peel. In addition, with the head elevated 45 degrees, there is less chance of the acid pooling around the eyes after it has been applied to the lower eyelid.

The acid can be applied to the skin with cotton-tipped applicators or 2×2 gauze squares. Because it is often necessary to rub the TCA into the skin, a brush is not an effective application device. I prefer using a 2×2 gauze sponge that has been folded into quarters because it allows me to rub the TCA into the skin. Attempting to rub the acid into the skin with a cotton-tipped applicator usually breaks the stick. I wet the folded 2×2 gauze with enough acid that two or three drops of TCA would drip off if it were squeezed. It is not dripping wet, nor is it squeezed dry.

I begin the application of the acid from the midline to the left side of the forehead, then from the midline to the right side of the forehead. I then apply the acid to the entire nose (Fig. 9-3). At this time, I stop the application to allow the patient to cool down and to give me the opportunity to observe the nature of the frost developing in the area where TCA has been applied. The second stage of application begins under the left eye, starting 2 to 3 mm below the lid margin and covering the entire left cheek and perioral area. Here, I again stop the application and watch the frost. The third stage is begun below the right eye and extends down the entire right cheek.

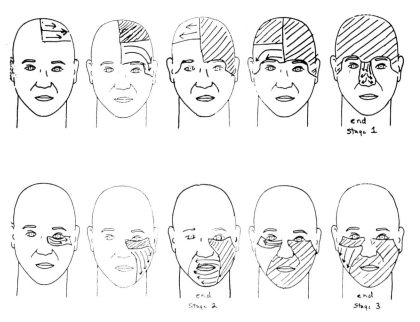

Figure 9-3
Diagram illustrating the three stages I use in the application of a TCA peel to the face.

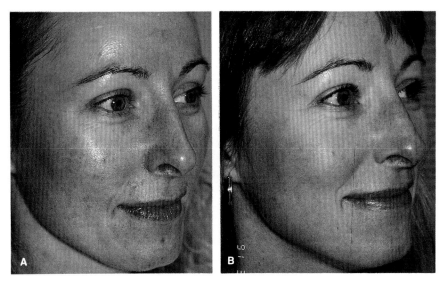

Figure 9-4

(*A*) A woman with level 1 photodamage. (*B*) The same woman 8 weeks after a level 2 TCA peel (using 30% TCA).

Several points should be addressed in regard to the application of the TCA:

1. The patient's head should be stabilized with one hand so you can press fairly hard with your gauze applicator as the acid is applied.
2. When applying the TCA below the eyes and in the "crow's feet" area, you must pull the surrounding skin tight so that
   a. the acid gets to the bottom of the wrinkle
   b. the wrinkle is temporarily stretched flat, preventing acid from being wicked into the eye along the wrinkle by capillary action
3. If you overlap coats of TCA, you will increase the depth of the peel. When using low strengths (less than 25% TCA), this is not much of a problem, but with higher concentrations, an area of accidental overlap can be a problem. Therefore, when applying TCA to the skin, always follow the same pattern of application, so you know where you have already applied the acid. In addition, it may be helpful to count the number of strokes you apply to each area to ensure the application of similar amounts of acid to all areas.
4. TCA peels work for photodamage (Fig. 9-4). There is rarely any photodamage on the upper eyelid, so there is no need to peel that area. However, the peel should be carried through the eyebrows to the edge of the upper orbital rim. Any excess drops of acid left on the eyebrow should be blotted off with a cotton-tipped applicator to prevent a deeper peel in the eyebrow area.

5. The peel should be carried into the hairline and 1 cm below the jawline to help blend the temporary pigmentation change associated with most peels.

As previously stated, it is imperative that you determine the peel depth required to appropriately treat the patient *before* beginning the peel. Interpreting acid penetration as you are performing the peel is crucial so that you know when the correct depth has been achieved. Fortunately, the depth of a TCA peel seems to correlate well with the intensity of the frost observed on the skin.

TCA is a chemical cauterant, which coagulates proteins in the skin. This is presumably the basis for the formation of the white frost seen when TCA is applied to the skin. The deeper the peel performed with TCA, the faster and more intensely white the frost. The intensity of the frost and its associated skin turgor are used to judge the depth of the peel. The levels of frost created by superficial and medium depth peels can be classified into four groups:

Level 0—no frost: The skin may look and feel a little slick and shiny, but there is no frost and minimal or no erythema. This is a very superficial peel that, at most, removes the stratum corneum.

Level 1—irregular light frost: In addition to appearing shiny, the skin shows some erythema and scattered areas of wispy white frost. This is a superficial epidermal peel that creates 2 to 4 days of light flaking (Fig. 9-5).

Level 2—white frost with pink showing through: The skin has a uniform white color but there is a strong pink background. This is a full-thickness epidermal peel that takes about 5 days to heal (Fig. 9-6).

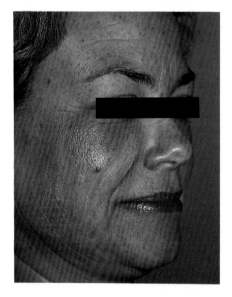

Figure 9-5
Level 1 TCA peel showing mild erythema with a wispy white frost.

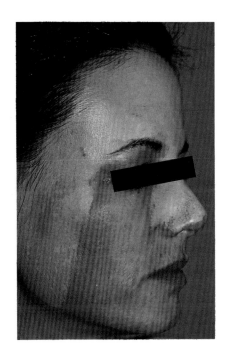

Figure 9-6

Level 2 TCA peel showing a uniform white frost with a prominent pink–red color still apparent in the background. (The entire face had not been peeled at the time of the photograph.)

> *Level 3—solid white frost:* The skin has a solid, intense white frost with no pink background showing through. This is a peel that extends into the papillary dermis and takes 5 to 7 days to heal (Fig. 9-7).

These levels of frost are guidelines; they vary a bit from patient to patient. However, they define a general pattern that is helpful in determining the depth of the wound that you have created.

In general, TCA in concentrations of 10% to 25% is used as an intraepidermal peeling agent; 30% to 40% is a papillary dermal peeling agent. The actual depth of penetration of the peeling agent is affected by many other variables, including type and thickness of the skin, degree and intensity of the skin priming, how the acid was applied to the skin, and how wet the acid applicator was. Therefore, it is always safest to use a lower concentration of TCA, so that if you fail to achieve as deep a peel as you want (you can judge this by examining the frost you created in the first area of your application), you can do several things to increase peel depth:

1. Apply a second coat of acid over the area that has already frosted (it is safest to decrease the strength of TCA in the second coat by 5% to 10% to prevent too deep a peel).

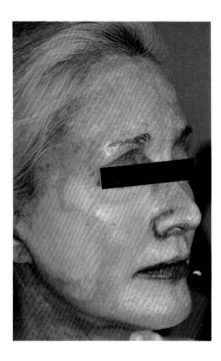

Figure 9-7

A woman with a level 2 TCA peel on most of her face, but several areas of level 3 peeling are apparent. A level 3 peel shows solid opaque white frost with no background erythema. These areas are most obvious in the preauricular area extending to the mid-cheek.

    2. When applying the TCA to the next (previously untreated) area on the face:

        a. Use a gauze sponge that is wetter. It will allow you to apply a greater quantity of acid, which will create a deeper peel.

        b. Rub the acid-soaked gauze more aggressively into the skin, trying to overlap areas of application.

Once the appropriate frost has been achieved, I often rinse the patient's face with room temperature water to wash off any excess acid that may remain on the skin. This does not "neutralize" the TCA; it dilutes any remaining reservoir of acid to prevent a deepening of the peel. (TCA is an aqueous solution, so adding water to it doesn't neutralize it—it dilutes it.)

Some physicians advocate applying ice packs to the skin after the peel to cool the skin and to decrease any residual burning. I have found most patients are hypersensitive immediately after the peel and that ice packs are too cold to be comfortable for them. Some patients don't even like the feeling of room temperature water applied to the skin at this time.

If you do apply water or ice compresses to the skin after a TCA peel, be sure to realize that you will have hydrated the stratum corneum and you cannot go back and reapply more TCA to this area because the acid will be rapidly diluted by the water trapped in the stratum corneum.

After the patient has washed his or her face and patted it dry, I apply a cream or an ointment with 1% hydrocortisone to soothe the skin. In theory, applying an occlusive ointment after the peel should function similarly to taping the skin after a peel. This has been shown to be true with phenol, for which applying petrolatum after a peel increases its penetration.

Occlusion

There is some degree of controversy as to whether taping a TCA peel increases or decreases its depth of penetration. There are two conflicting studies at this time, so no one knows the answer. Since I began using an ointment postpeel, I have not noticed any unexpected results from peels that would indicate increased or decreased penetration.

Postpeel Care

Patients can and should expect certain things while healing from a TCA peel (Fig. 9-8):

1. The skin will look and feel tight, as if it were covered with a sheet of plastic.
2. Any area of epidermal hyperpigmentation will darken considerably as part of its reaction to the peel.
3. Varying degrees of erythema may be present, often in a blotchy, uneven distribution.
4. Varying degrees of swelling can occur. It is rare to see such edema with superficial peels, but some edema is common with papillary dermal peels. The edema usually peaks 48 hours after the peel.
5. The first areas to begin peeling will be the areas with the most muscle movement (ie, perioral and periorbital areas).
6. The forehead and hairline are usually the last areas to peel.

The layer of necrotic, peeled tissue protects the underlying new tissue. Premature removal of any of this layer increases the risk of persistent erythema, infection, postinflammatory hyperpigmentation and scarring. Therefore, the goal of postpeel care is to keep this layer of tissue in place as long as possible and to keep patients comfortable so they will not be tempted to pick or scratch at their skin.

It is helpful to tell patients to try not to have any shear forces against their skin, which can create premature peeling. This means a special approach to washing the face and applying emollients:

Washing: Always use a mild soap like Purpose or Neutrogena, or a soap-free cleanser like Cetaphil. The patient should gently splash lukewarm water on the face, then lather soap on his or her hands and pat the

(text continues on p. 124)

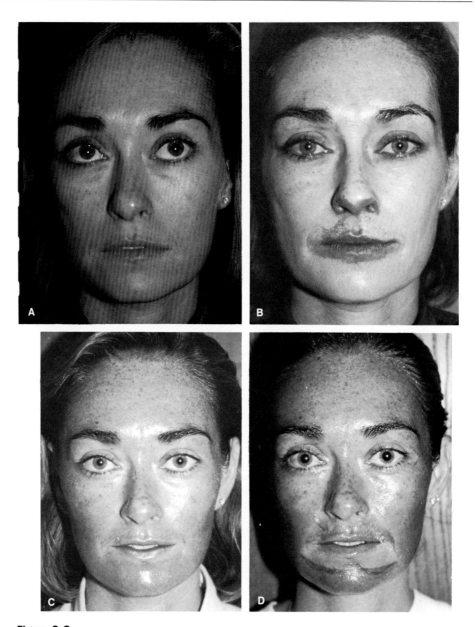

Figure 9-8

Daily photographs of a 30-year-old patient healing during a level 2 TCA peel. (*A*) Before the peel, the patient displays level 1 photodamage. (*B*) Five minutes after the application of 30% TCA to create a level 2 peel. (*C*) One day after the peel, all areas of previous pigmentation have darkened. (*D*) Two days afterward, the perioral area is beginning to peel. (*E*) At 3 days, the skin is continuing to peel from the central face outward. (*F*) Four days postpeel. (*G*) Five days afterward, persistent areas of peeling skin still present along hairline. (*H*) Seven days after the peel, the skin has a clear, freshened appearance.

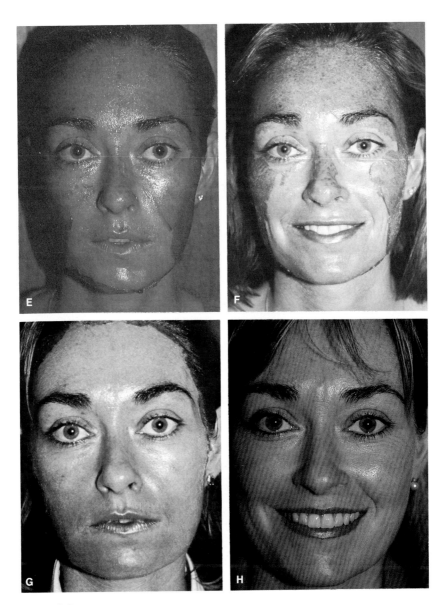

Figure 9-8   (Continued)

lather onto the skin. The lather is then rinsed off and the face gently patted dry with a soft towel. **It is not necessary to try to wash off all remnants of the previously applied emollients.**

Applying emollients: When applying any cream or ointment, every effort should be made to *pat* rather than rub the product onto the skin. Since this is particularly hard to do with most ointments (they usually are stiff), it is helpful to put a dab of ointment in the palm of the hand and allow it to warm up and liquefy before applying it to the skin.

STRICT RULES FOR PATIENTS DURING THE HEALING PHASE

▶ Avoid all sun exposure.
▶ Avoid exercise and sweating.
▶ Avoid having the shower spray strike directly on your face.
▶ Do not pick, rub, or unnecessarily touch your face.
▶ Minimize facial expression.
▶ Try to sleep on your back (this is particularly important for medium depth peels).
▶ If you shampoo your hair, it should be done with your head tilted backward into the sink so no soap runs down your face.

Depending on the level of the TCA peel, the wound care can vary a good deal:

Very superficial intraepidermal peels: The patient should expect some tightness and perhaps mild erythema with associated flaking for 2 to 4 days. During this time, the use of a bland emollient is encouraged. The patient can wear makeup and is allowed to shower, but must avoid rubbing his or her face.

Superficial, full-thickness epidermal peels: This level of peel turns dark and unsightly for 4 to 6 days. The skin becomes extremely tight and will fissure and crack if it is not moist enough. These patients normally do not go to work and are unable to wear makeup. I prefer that they do not shower or swim since it seems to create premature peeling. The use of bland emollients is acceptable for these patients, but their skin is so dry that they need to reapply cream every 1 to 2 hours. Therefore, some patients prefer to use a greasier product, like an ointment. Your choices here include polysporin, bacitracin, petrolatum, vegetable shortening, and 1% hydrocortisone ointment (see section on wound healing).

It is important to keep the skin of these patients moisturized while healing. If it becomes too dry, it may crack, exposing the immature layer of skin. In addition, dry skin has a tendency to become itchy, which increases the chances patients will pick or rub it.

Papillary dermal peels: This level of peel turns dark and unsightly for 5 to 8 days. There is often some mild swelling (particularly in the periorbital area) for the first 48 hours postpeel. Some patients, particularly those with a history of previous facial surgery or of severe sun damage, experience marked edema of the lower two thirds of their face, which can last 3 or 4 days. This is fairly uncommon and can be helped by sleeping with the head elevated. Ice compresses should be avoided, since they have a tendency to traumatize the peeling skin or to overhydrate it (from the condensation on the outside of the ice packs).

This level of peel feels rather tight for most of the healing phase, and most patients are more comfortable with the use of ointments several times a day. My preference is 1% hydrocortisone ointment because it decreases the itching and irritation often associated with these peels.

Patients with papillary dermal peels are quite unattractive while healing. They are unable to wear makeup, and most stay in the home. They often feel a bit fatigued during their healing phase, and they should be encouraged to try to rest and relax as much as possible.

Compresses

The use of compresses during the healing phase is a matter of personal preference. They are rarely, if ever, necessary for superficial peels. However, some physicians believe they speed up healing with medium depth peels.

Normally, I use compresses whenever there are any areas of a peel that look necrotic or exudative. The compress serves to desiccate this juicy tissue, thereby creating an environment poorly conducive to bacterial growth. If the compress contains 3% hydrogen peroxide or 0.25% acetic acid, it will also have an antibacterial effect, which can be helpful.

▷ Nonfacial Peels With Trichloroacetic Acid

The techniques for nonfacial peels with TCA are exactly the same as for facial peels. However, care must be taken to avoid performing a dermal peel in these areas, since they scar so easily. Therefore, the end point of this nonfacial TCA peel is a level 2 frost (Fig. 9-9). Remember, although this is an epidermal peel, repeated treatments can create new collagen deposition in the dermis and may be able to improve some fine wrinkles (Fig. 9-10).

Because an accidental dermal peel of nonfacial skin can be a disaster, it is safest to start peeling nonfacial areas with low levels of TCA (20% to 25%). It may be necessary to apply several coats to achieve the level of frost you desire, but this is much safer than starting with too high a concentration of acid and accidentally creating a deep peel.

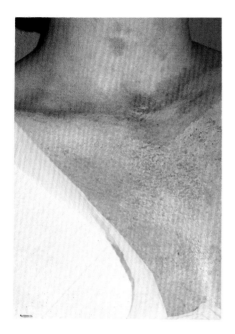

Figure 9-9
Level 2 TCA frost on the chest. There is uniform whiteness with a strong red background showing through.

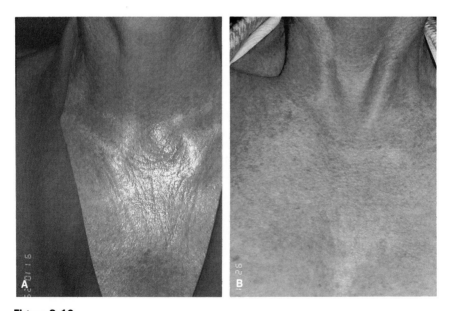

Figure 9-10
(*A*) A woman with fine vertical wrinkling in the presternal area. (*B*) The same patient 2 months after two level 2 TCA peels.

▷ Enhanced or Combination Peels

Over the years, several ways of enhancing the penetration of an acid have been devised. I have already discussed the effect of priming and cleaning the skin in relation to the depth of the peel. In this section, I will examine the effects of combining two peeling or wounding agents in an effort to create a deeper peel. This concept is of particular concern in regard to TCA. Because most physicians think that high concentrations of TCA (over 40% to 50%) are more apt to create scarring, the goal of combination peels is to be able to use a lower concentration of TCA (35%) but have it penetrate as deeply as 50% TCA.

The most commonly used combination peels are as follows:

- ▶ Jessner's solution and TCA
- ▶ Solid carbon dioxide and TCA
- ▶ Glycolic acid and TCA
- ▶ Jessner's solution and glycolic acid

Jessner's Solution and TCA

This peel combination has been popularized by Dr. Gary Monheit. With this technique, the patient is primed and the skin cleaned in the usual manner. Then, one to four layers of Jessner's solution are applied to the face—with the end point being a fairly uniform erythema with areas of light frost. Remember to wait about 5 minutes between application of the Jessner's solution to allow it to penetrate before applying any more solution.

After the Jessner's solution has penetrated into the skin, TCA 35% is applied in the usual manner. Since the Jessner's solution disrupts the barrier function of the skin, the TCA penetrates more rapidly and uniformly than if it were applied on untreated skin. Histologic studies have shown that the depth of the combination peel is greater than with TCA 35% alone, and there is evidence of new collagen deposition from this combination peel. You can use this combination with other strengths of TCA, but caution must be used if you use TCA 40% to 50% because you will create a much deeper peel.

In patients with thick, sebaceous skin, the application of several coats of Jessner's solution before applying the TCA allows a deeper, more uniform peel. However, in patients with drier or thinner skin, there may be no reason to perform this type of combination peel.

Drawbacks

1. Jessner's solution stings and burns. If you apply two or three coats of it before you apply the TCA, the patient will be more sensitive and uncomfortable when you apply the TCA.

2. It takes 5 to 10 minutes to apply one coat of a Jessner's solution and to evaluate it. So if you apply three coats of Jessner's solution before performing the TCA peel, it may take you an additional 15 to 30 minutes to do the procedure.

Solid Carbon Dioxide and TCA

This peel has been popularized by Dr. Hal Brody. He has studied it and written about it extensively and has shown that it creates a significantly deeper peel than TCA alone or even the combined Jessner's solution and TCA peel.

With this technique, the patient is primed and the skin cleaned in the usual manner. A block of solid carbon dioxide (dry ice) is broken into a handheld size and is dipped into a solution of three parts acetone to one part alcohol. (This allows the solid carbon dioxide to glide over the skin without sticking.) The solid carbon dioxide is then applied to areas of the face where you want the peel to penetrate deeper (eg, over a wrinkle, along the rim of the scar). The more pressure that is exerted when applying the solid carbon dioxide to the skin, the deeper the wound it creates. Brody uses mild (3 to 5 seconds), moderate (5 to 8 seconds) and hard (8 to 15 seconds) as his classification system.

After applying the solid carbon dioxide, the skin is wiped dry; when the stinging induced by the carbon dioxide subsides, TCA 35% (or other concentrations) can then be applied to the face in the usual manner. Because the areas treated with solid carbon dioxide and TCA sustain a deeper wound, they will heal a little more slowly than the rest of the face.

Drawbacks

1. Solid carbon dioxide is difficult to store in the office (although it is easy to get a block of it from an ice cream store on the day of the peel).
2. Moderate or hard pressure with solid carbon dioxide can be quite uncomfortable to many patients, and they may not want you to freeze any other areas after you have treated the first two or three.

Glycolic Acid and TCA

This peel was recently presented by Dr. William Coleman. The concept of this peel, like the two peels previously discussed, is to achieve a more uniform, deeper peel than with TCA alone. Coleman's data suggest that this combination does penetrate a bit deeper than TCA alone, and he believes it to be a more uniform peel.

With this technique, the patient is primed in the usual manner, but the skin is not cleaned. Glycolic acid 70% is applied to the face for 2 minutes and then washed off with water. Next, TCA 35% is applied in the usual manner.

Drawbacks

1. The addition of a glycolic acid peel to the TCA peel creates new collagen deposition in the upper dermis. However, at this time, there has been no comparison of combined glycolic acid and TCA peels versus TCA peels alone to show whether the combination peel is any more effective than TCA alone.
2. Glycolic acid peels are uneven. It seems dangerous to create an uneven wound and then immediately follow it with a more caustic peeling agent. Common sense would dictate that this should create a very uneven TCA peel.
3. When you perform and neutralize a glycolic acid peel, you are applying water to the stratum corneum, which may dilute the TCA immediately applied to the skin after the glycolic acid peel.

Jessner's Solution and Glycolic Acid

This peel combination has been popularized by Dr. Larry Moy. There are two ideas behind this peel:

▶ The Jessner's solution disrupts the barrier function of the skin, allowing the glycolic acid to create a more uniform depth peel.
▶ Jessner's solution normally creates exfoliation of the skin, whereas glycolic acid may not. So, the use of both agents together gives the patient the immediate benefits of exfoliation as well as some of the slower stimulatory benefits of a glycolic acid peel.

With this technique, the patient is primed and the skin is cleaned in the usual manner. One to three coats of Jessner's solution are applied to the skin until the end point of diffuse, mild erythema is reached. Then glycolic acid 70% is applied and left on the skin until an increase in erythema is noted. The glycolic acid is then neutralized.

Drawbacks

1. It is a risky peel to perform since the patient's skin is already red before you apply the glycolic acid. It is easy to overpeel the patient and create areas of epidermolysis.
2. There are no histologic studies showing any increased efficacy of this peel over either Jessner's peels or glycolic acid peels alone.

Manual of Chemical Peels: Superficial and Medium Depth, by Mark G. Rubin.
J.B. Lippincott Company, Philadelphia, © 1995.

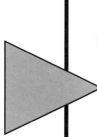

CHAPTER **10**

COMPLICATIONS

Tears Dripping Onto the Neck ▸ *Premature
Peeling* ▸ *Infection* ▸ *Acneform Eruptions* ▸
Ecchymoses ▸ *Postinflammatory Hyperpigmentation* ▸
Hypopigmentation ▸ *Allergic Reactions* ▸
Persistent Erythema ▸ *Scarring*

It is an unfortunate but undeniable truth of chemical peeling that some patients
will experience complications. The key to successful chemical peeling is to minimize the possible complications. If, despite your best efforts, a complication
develops, rapid and appropriate treatment is usually able to correct the complication without an unacceptable cosmetic outcome.

The adage, "The best defense is a good offense," is an appropriate reminder
that the best way to minimize complications is to avoid performing peels on those
at risk for complications, such as the following:

▸ Patients with histories of poor wound healing and keloid formation
▸ Patients with histories of postinflammatory hyperpigmentation
▸ Patients who are unable or unwilling to stay out of the sun
▸ Patients who fail to follow instructions
▸ Patients with histories of extremely sensitive skin that is easily irritated
  by most skin care products

There is no reason that these patients cannot be peeled. They are a high-risk
group, however, and you may wish to avoid peeling them or you may opt to use a
lighter peel. Remember, the deeper the peel, the greater the risk of complications.
Intraepidermal peels have markedly fewer complications than reticular dermal
peels. Therefore, when performing a peel on a patient at risk for a complication,
you may choose to do several lighter peels rather than one deep one in an effort to
produce improvement with little risk of complications.

The most common complications with a chemical peel are

▶ tears dripping onto the neck
▶ premature peeling
▶ infection
▶ acneform eruptions
▶ ecchymosis
▶ postinflammatory hyperpigmentation
▶ hypopigmentation
▶ allergic reactions
▶ persistent erythema
▶ scarring

▷ Tears Dripping Onto the Neck

Whenever a caustic substance is applied around the eyes or nose, the reflex action is to develop tears. This is a normal, acceptable reflex helpful in preventing ocular damage if any acid were to get into the eye. A dry eye is unable to dilute the concentration of an acid coming into contact with the eye, whereas the aqueous solution in a tearing eye instantly dilutes the acid, making it less caustic.

Tearing of the eyes causes two primary problems:

1. Tears can drip down the cheeks and dilute the acid still on the cheeks, causing a strip of skin where the peel is more superficial.
2. Tears can drip down the cheek, mixing with the acid there, and continue to drip down onto the neck, causing an area of peeling on the neck (Fig. 10-1). This can be a particularly severe problem if the concentration of acid is high, since the neck is more easily prone to scarring. I have seen tears carry trichloroacetic acid 50% (TCA) onto the neck and create a hypertrophic scar.

A patient is often unable to notice when his or her eyes are tearing during the peel. Therefore, it is important to have someone watch the patient's eyes closely during the peel and to dry any tears before they roll down the cheek. This is best done by dabbing the tear with a cotton-tipped applicator. It is also possible to put a protective layer of petrolatum on the neck before the peel to guard against any accidental burns on the neck. I recommend against the use of a topical anesthetic in the eye to decrease tearing, since some degree of tearing is helpful to protect the eye from a burn if acid inadvertently gets in the eye.

If tearing occurs and an obvious strip of lesser peeling is seen on the cheek, additional peeling agent can be applied to that area after drying the tear. If the acid-containing tear drips onto the neck, the area should be washed with water to dilute any remaining TCA and then treated like any other postpeel area with daily wound care.

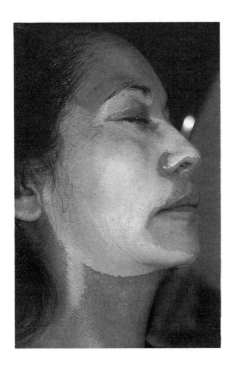

Figure 10-1

While this patient was undergoing a level 3 TCA peel, a tear ran from her right eye, down her cheek, and onto her neck. The tear carried some TCA onto the neck, where it created a linear area of peeling.

▷ Premature Peeling

Premature peeling can be a problem with any level of peel. The layer of necrotic skin created by the peeling solution functions as a protective bandage, allowing the deeper tissue to heal before being exposed to the elements at the skin surface. Premature removal of this layer, accidental or intentional, exposes a layer of immature tissue that is fragile and possibly not reepithelialized. This can lead to infection, persistent erythema, postinflammatory hyperpigmentation, and scarring.

Although patients generally do not plan on picking at their peeling skin, most do, usually during the last few days of the peel when they are tired of the peeling process and want to accelerate it. Common hallmarks of premature peeling are

▶ sharply demarcated areas of bright erythema (Fig. 10-2)
▶ a peel that is completed within 24 to 48 hours of being only halfway finished
▶ no evidence of old peeling skin anywhere on the face, including the hairline (most patients have small areas of peeling skin in the hairline for 8 to 10 days after a peel)

Areas of premature peeling commonly present either as non-reepithelialized tissue or bright red reepithelialized skin.

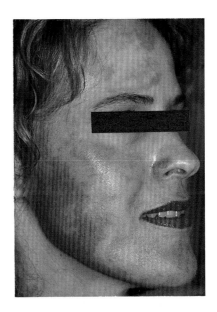

Figure 10-2

A woman 5 days after a level 2 TCA peel. During healing, she picked off some of the peeling skin. The sharply demarcated area of bright erythema on her left lateral cheek corresponds to the area of premature peeling.

Non-Reepithelialized Tissue

In areas in which the peeled skin was removed before the underlying tissue had a chance to reepithelialize, the tissue may look raw or fairly normal but moist and succulent (Fig. 10-3). The first priority in areas of non-reepithelialized tissue is to get the skin to heal and to prevent infections. Aggressive wound care management with the application of topical antibiotics (Polysporin, Bacitracin, Bactroban, Silvadene) four times a day is usually all that is needed.

Reepithelialization can be enhanced with the use of Vigilon, a hydrocolloid dressing applied twice daily to the wound. One layer of the plastic film is removed, and the exposed gel is applied directly to the wound. Unfortunately, the Vigilon must be taped to the skin to be held in place. This usually can be accomplished with paper tape. However, if the surrounding skin has not peeled yet, it is impossible to tape the Vigilon in place and it cannot be used.

An open wound is an invitation to infection, so I always place patients with areas of non-reepithelialized skin on regimens of oral antibiotics with *Staphylococcus* and *Streptococcus* coverage (eg, cephalosporins, erythromycins, sulfa drugs—all of which work well) until reepithelialization is complete.

Reepithelialized, Bright Red Tissue

Reepithelialized but bright red tissue is healed over, so there is no risk of infection, but it is paper-thin and very fragile. The patient must be instructed to care for this skin as if it were the skin of a newborn baby just home from the hospital.

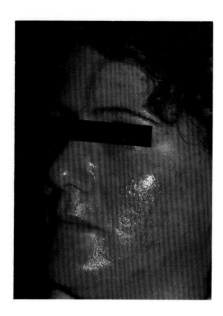

Figure 10-3

A woman 4 days after a level 2 TCA peel. During healing, she picked off all areas of peeling skin. The skin on her cheeks appears brightly erythematous and "juicy" where it is not completely reepithelialized.

No mechanical trauma, including rubbing, is allowed, and a protective layer of an ointment must be applied several times a day.

The potential problems with these areas are postinflammatory hyperpigmentation and persistent erythema, both of which are considered later in this chapter. The goal is to prevent the development of these problems by stopping the inflammation before it progresses into a complication.

Patients with reepithelialized, bright red tissue are usually a tender, itchy, or sensitive in these inflamed areas. To decrease inflammation, you can use topical corticosteroids, Catrix cream, oral nonsteroidal antiinflammatory drugs (NSAIDs), or systemic steroids. The oral NSAIDs are usually not particularly helpful in these patients. Although systemic steroids can be effective, it is usually best to try topical therapies first, since they have less risk of complications.

When a topical cortisone is to be applied to inflamed skin, the product's base is important. Products with enhanced delivery systems (including propylene glycol) are often irritating to this sensitive skin. As a general rule, ointments are more soothing than creams for the following reasons:

1. They create a better protective barrier than a cream.
2. They have fewer chemical additives.
3. They enhance the penetration of the cortisone.

However, ointments are often unpleasant for patients to wear on the face because it is difficult, if not impossible, to apply makeup on top of an ointment. Because reepithelialized, bright red tissue usually is a complication more than 1 week after a peel, these patients often need to be back functioning in society at this time. For

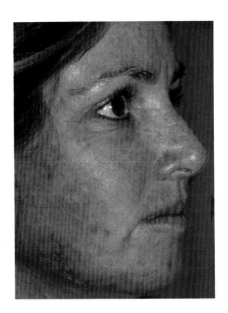

Figure 10-4
Early infection with *Staphylococcus aureus* along the right jawline 7 days after a level 3 TCA peel.

this reason, I often prescribe a cream with a bland base, the least irritating of which are Locoid cream and DesOwen cream.

The erythema usually improves dramatically within 4 to 7 days. If it fails to improve during this time, I increase the strength of the cortisone creams to a class III topical steroid like Topicort cream or Aristocort A (neither has propylene glycol or parabens, both of which can be sensitizers). Although class III topical steroids are generally considered too strong for the face, 5 to 7 days of use should not cause any problems.

▷ Infection

Fortunately, infections associated with chemical peels are infrequent. As a rule, the incidence of infection increases with the depth of the peel. This is due in part to the fact that peels that form crusts (deep peels) are more prone to bacterial colonization, leading to infection, than are peels that do not form crusts.

Because infections commonly lead to scarring, any suspicion of infection should be treated aggressively. Infections appear to significantly deepen the wound induced by the peeling agent, so rapid treatment intervention is needed to achieve a satisfactory cosmetic outcome.

Several organisms can create the infections associated with peels:

▶ Common bacterial pathogens—*Staphylococcus* and *Streptococcus* species (Fig. 10-4)

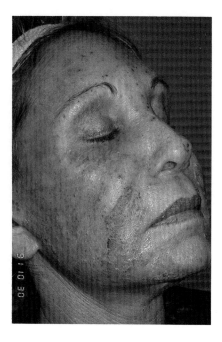

Figure 10-5

Pseudomonas aeruginosa infection in the right nasolabial area 5 days after a level 2 TCA peel.

▶ Uncommon bacterial pathogens—*Pseudomonas* and *Enterobacter* species (Fig. 10-5)
▶ Herpes simplex
▶ *Candida* species (Fig. 10-6)

The presentations of early infections with any of these organisms can be strikingly similar. Therefore, a bacterial culture should be taken from any suspicious area. In addition, a Gram stain can provide some useful information rapidly (eg, candidiasis versus gram-positive or gram-negative bacteria).

It is helpful to put the patient on a broad-spectrum oral antibiotic regimen that covers both gram-positive and gram-negative organisms while you await the culture results. I routinely use ofloxacin (Floxin), 400 mg twice a day. After the culture and sensitivity results are back, a more specific oral antibiotic can be prescribed.

Appropriate topical wound care of infected areas is vital. Mupirocin ointment (Bactroban) or gentamicine ointment (Garamycin) applied four times a day can be helpful both for the positive effect on wound healing of the base and for antibacterial action (Bactroban for *Staphylococcus* and *Streptococcus*; Garamycin for *Staphylococcus*, *Streptococcus*, and some gram-negative organisms).

If crusted or necrotic debris is seen on the wound, it must be removed with compresses or gentle mechanical debridement. Compresses containing 0.25% to 0.5% acetic acid are especially effective against gram-negative bacteria. Gentle mechanical debridement either can be performed by you or your staff in the office

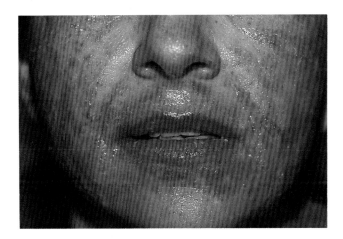

Figure 10-6

Candida infection in a patient 5 days after a level 3 TCA peel. White plaques (thrush) are visible on the lips.

or can be accomplished at home by the patient's standing in the shower and letting water run down his or her face (not striking the face directly).

If the patient has a candidal infection, treatment with oral ketoconazole (Nizoral), 200 mg per day, is highly effective. In addition, using wet to dry compresses containing distilled water or saline twice a day helps to create an environment less conducive to growth of *Candida* organisms.

Herpetic outbreaks, usually starting on the lip or above the vermillion border, can be triggered by the trauma of a chemical peel. Since the peeling skin does not have a well-developed epidermis, it is not capable of forming a vesicle. Therefore, herpetic infections in peeling patients present with erosions rather than vesicles. The one cardinal sign of herpetic infection is pain. Therefore, as Brody states, "Any painful lesions is herpes until proven otherwise." With the use of prophylactic oral acyclovir (Zoviraz), 400 mg three times a day, herpetic outbreaks are rarely a problem. However, occasional patients with no history of herpes labialis may experience outbreaks. These are patients who had been previously infected but had forgotten or were unaware. These patients need immediate oral acyclovir, 400 mg three to four times a day, as well as topical acyclovir applied to the area six times a day. On rare occasions, a patient may not respond well to this dosage, usually because of poor absorption of the drug. In these cases, increase the dose of acyclovir to 400 mg five times a day.

In summary, the key points about infections are as follows:

1. Superficial and medium depth peels should not create heavy crusts. Assume any area of crusting is an incipient infection and treat appropriately.
2. Perform a culture and Gram stain of any suspicious area. This will identify bacteria and candidal organisms.
3. Look along the lips and on the oral mucosa for signs of thrush.

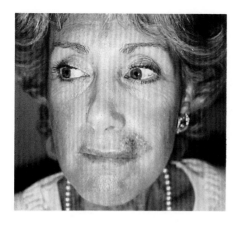

Figure 10-7
A contact dermatitis to Bacitracin ointment above the patient's left upper lip 8 days after a level 2 TCA peel.

4. Assume any painful lesion is herpes until proved otherwise, even in patients who do not remember a prior episode of herpes simplex or who do not present with vesicles.
5. Treat all infections aggressively with oral and topical antibiotics.
6. If an area fails to grow anything on cultures and continues to worsen despite treatment, consider the possibility of a contact dermatitis to one of the topical agents (Fig. 10-7).

Acneform Eruptions

A small percentage of patients experience acneform eruptions during or just after the peeling phase (Fig. 10-8). This condition usually appears as multiple tender erythematous follicular papules. These lesions are different from the superficial pustules that can be seen during the healing stage of a peel, which are secondary to follicular occlusion from the emollients and ointments used during the healing phase. True acneform eruptions rarely show pustules and are almost always tender to touch. They respond promptly to antibiotic therapy used to treat normal acne—that is, topical clindamycin or erythromycin, as well as systemic tetracycline, minocycline, or erythromycin. It usually takes 5 to 10 days for acneform eruptions to clear completely.

▷ Ecchymoses

A small number of patients may develop ecchymoses in the infraorbital area associated with their peel (Fig. 10-9). This is seen only in patients who have pronounced swelling in this area during the healing phase of the peel. Generally,

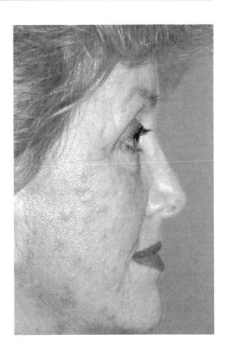

Figure 10-8
Acneform eruption, characterized by tender erythematous papules 7 days after a level 3 TCA peel.

these patients have significant actinic damage and marked atrophy of the skin. Presumably, the periorbital edema causes a rupture in some of the small vessels of the dermal plexus, creating an ecchymosis. Interestingly, this complication is no more common in patients taking NSAIDs or warfarin (Coumadin) than in those taking no medications.

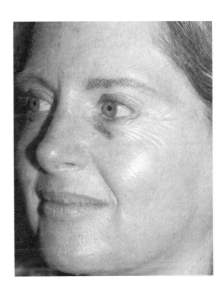

Figure 10-9
An ecchymosis in the left infraorbital area 10 days after a level 3 TCA peel.

Ecchymoses are a self-limited complication that has no negative impact on the final result of the peel. Conceptually, it would be possible to develop some residual hyperpigmentation secondary to hemosiderin deposition, but I have never seen this happen.

The treatment for ecchymoses is reassurance and the use of camouflage makeup if needed. The discoloration should resolve completely within 4 to 6 weeks.

▷ Postinflammatory Hyperpigmentation

Postinflammatory hyperpigmentation is a condition in which an inflammatory response of the skin leads to the development of subsequent hyperpigmentation (Fig. 10-10). Classically, this has been described as being associated with dark-skinned patients, but it can also occur (with lesser frequency) in patients with light skin and light eyes.

Some authorities have stated that this condition is always triggered by excessive sun exposure after a peel, but I have seen this in patients who have had no postpeel sun exposure at all. Certainly, the underlying tendency for this type of hyperpigmentation seems to be innate in most people who have it. It is rare to see postinflammatory hyperpigmentation after a peel in a patient who has no history of it from other inflammatory conditions. Therefore, it is helpful to question such patients about their tendency to display hyperpigmentation from minor trauma like cuts or insect bites before performing the peel. If a patient has this tendency, you know there is a high chance that he or she will experience hyperpigmentation from any peel that creates significant inflammation.

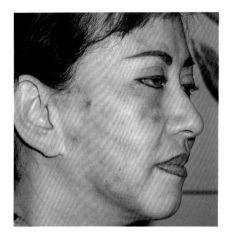

Figure 10-10

Postinflammatory hyperpigmentation in an Asian patient 3 weeks after a level 2 TCA peel.

When dealing with postinflammatory hyperpigmentation, several key points should be kept in mind:

1. Postinflammatory hyperpigmentation will gradually improve with time with no therapy except sun avoidance.
2. Epidermal postinflammatory hyperpigmentation responds well to a variety of therapies, but dermal postinflammatory hyperpigmentation does not respond so uniformly well.
3. Postinflammatory hyperpigmentation is initiated (and can be worsened) by inflammation. Therefore, all efforts at reducing it must also try to eliminate inflammation.

Postinflammatory hyperpigmentation can develop as quickly as 4 or 5 days after a peel or as long as 2 months afterward. Therefore, when peeling patients at risk for this condition, you must be an astute observer for their entire course of healing.

Treatment

Sunscreen.   Because postinflammatory hyperpigmentation is worsened by ultraviolet (UV) light, daily use of broad-spectrum sunscreens is mandatory. UVA light passes through glass, so the patient needs to block this type of light each day, even if rarely outside. Some evidence even suggests that long-wavelength UVA light can be emitted by certain types of fluorescent light, meaning patients who are never outside may still be at risk for hyperpigmentation if exposed to fluorescent light.

The best sunscreen to use would be a physical blocking sunscreen, but most patients are unwilling to wear these because of their thick, heavy appearance. Certainly, broad-spectrum sunscreens with both UVA- and UVB-blocking chemicals are helpful at screening out a large percentage of UV light. However, none of these cosmetically elegant products are total blocks. Therefore, wearing a hat or visor in addition to the sunscreen is advisable whenever possible.

Determination of the depth of pigmentation.   Always examine the skin using a Wood's lamp. Epidermal pigmentation is accentuated with this light, and dermal pigmentation is deaccentuated. In simpler terms, the more apparent the pigmentation is when viewed with a Wood's lamp, the more superficial the pigmentation. Remember, epidermal hyperpigmentation responds much better to treatment than does dermal hyperpigmentation.

Bleaching agents.   We really have no true bleaching agents to use on the skin. The most commonly used chemicals in the treatment of hyperpigmentation are actually tyrosinase inhibitors, which prevent the conversion of tyrosine to dopa. These chemicals decrease the skin's ability to manufacture melanin, thereby creating a gradual lightening effect.

At this time, the most commonly used tyrosinase inhibitors are hydroquinone, kojic acid, and azelaic acid. In the United States, hydroquinone is by far the most commonly used bleaching agent, whereas kojic acid is popular in the Far East and azelaic acid is popular in parts of Europe. It is important to realize that none of these products is tremendously effective. The best results are obtained by combining a tyrosine inhibitor with another product that has its own bleaching effect, enhances the penetration of the bleaching agent, or stimulates epidermal growth, thereby accelerating epidermal cell shedding. Because epidermal cells contain melanin, increasing their shedding decreases the total amount of melanin present in the epidermis, creating less pigmentation and a lightening effect. The most commonly used products to improve the efficacy of a bleaching agent are retinoic acid (Retin A) and alpha hydroxy acids (AHAs).

The standard enhanced bleaching routine has been the Kligman formula, which is made of a combination of 0.1% retinoic acid cream, 4% hydroquinone, and triamcinolone acetonide. Clinical studies have shown that the steroid is not necessary for the bleaching effect. It has also been shown that using hydroquinone in concentrations higher than 4% is more effective but significantly more irritating to the skin.

It has been my experience during the past 3 or 4 years that the combination of 10% glycolic acid with 4% hydroquinone is far superior to the combination of 0.1% retinoic acid cream and 4% hydroquinone. In addition to its improved efficacy, this combination also has the benefits of not inducing erythema, scaling, inflammation, or photosensitivity (as is often the case with mixtures of retinoic acid and hydroquinone).

Recently, another bleaching agent has proved even more effective than the glycolic acid and hydroquinone mixture. The new product is made up of 3% citric acid, 3% lactic acid mixed with 2% hydroquinone and 2% kojic acid. Presumably, there is a synergistic effect between several of these agents, since this is a highly effective product despite the bleaching agents that are present in low concentrations.

Any bleaching agent should be applied to the hyperpigmented areas twice a day. Some degree of clinical improvement should be seen in 3 to 4 weeks, but maximal results take 2 to 3 months.

Repeeling. If the patient's postinflammatory hyperpigmentation is responding slowly to the use of the bleachers and sunscreens, a superficial peel can accelerate the response. The goal of this type of peel is to exfoliate some of the epidermal cells (containing melanin) without creating enough inflammation to trigger another case of postinflammatory hyperpigmentation. This type of peel can be performed with 10% TCA, Jessner's solution, or 50% to 70% glycolic acid. These should be *conservative* peels. It is safer to perform very light exfoliations every 10 to 14 days than to peel too deeply, which can recreate postinflammatory hyperpigmentation. **Although light peels are an excellent way of treating postinflammatory hyperpigmentation, many patients with hyperpigmentation due to a peel are not eager to undergo repeeling.**

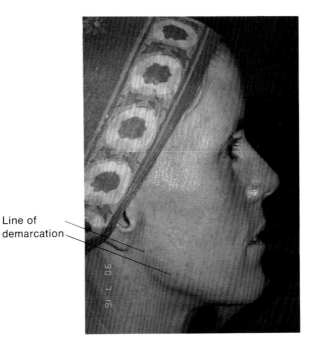

Line of
demarcation

Figure 10-11

Transient hypopigmentation of the face
10 days after a level 2 TCA peel. The
line of demarcation along the jawline
should resolve completely within 2 or 3
months.

▷ Hypopigmentation

Any peel that causes actual peeling or exfoliation will lighten the skin. Because melanin is dispersed (in melanosomes) throughout the epidermis, if you shed some cells containing melanin, the total amount of melanin present in the epidermis is reduced, creating a lighter appearance. However, lightening is transient since new melanin is continually formed.

As the level of the peel gets deeper, the degree of lightening or hypopigmentation increases. Remember that melanin is created in melanocytes, which are dispersed along the basal cell layer of the epidermis and extend down the hair follicle. If you remove the entire epidermis, including the basal cell layer, the melanocytes available to migrate into the new epidermis are those in the hair follicle. It takes several months for these melanocytes to effectively repopulate the new epidermis and give it a normal color. Therefore, a patient undergoing a full-thickness epidermal peel will have some degree of hypopigmentation for at least 2 or 3 months (Fig. 10-11).

As the depth of the peel increases, more melanocytes in the hair follicle are damaged or destroyed, leading to greater degrees of hypopigmentation. Also, as more melanocytes are destroyed, an increasing percentage of the resultant hypopigmentation becomes irreversible. Reticular dermal peeling with any peeling agent always creates some degree of permanent hypopigmentation (Fig. 10-12). However, with deeper peels, repigmentation of the peeled skin can take up to 3 years to reach its maximum.

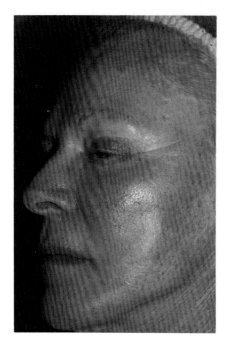

Figure 10-12
Persistent patchy hypopigmentation in a woman 2 years
after a deep reticular dermal TCA peel.

When dealing with hypopigmentation, there are two key points to keep in mind:

1. If the patient is using retinoic acid, AHA, hydroquinone, or sunscreen on the face but not the neck, he or she will always be hypopigmented on the face relative to the neck. Therefore, it is important in any peel that wounds the basal cell layer or deeper to apply retinoic acid, AHA, hydroquinone, or sunscreen to the neck as well as the face. This will help prevent a line of demarcation in color. It seems obvious, but many people fail to realize that tanning the neck while protecting the face (with sunscreen) makes the face appear lighter. It is your responsibility to tell the patient to apply sunscreen, as well as postpeel maintenance products, to the upper neck as well as the face.
2. Most adults who have actinic damage of the face also have some degree of permanent hyperpigmentation on their skin. It may be obvious on the rest of the body as a permanent "tan line" from a bathing suit or may be visible only on the face and neck with the use of a Wood's lamp. (Shine a Wood's lamp on the sun-damaged lateral side of the neck, and contrast it with the sun-spared area directly under the chin.)

When you remove the damaged epidermis and replace it with a new epidermis, the new skin is really the color of the normal non–sun-damaged skin. It is not necessarily hypopigmented, just as the skin on the volar forearm is lighter than the skin on the dorsal forearm but is not considered hypopigmented. Therefore, any peel that improves sun damage will make the skin a little lighter because healthy skin is lighter than sun-damaged skin. However, this degree of lightening should be slight enough not to be a cosmetic liability in most cases of nonphenol medium depth peels.

▷ Allergic Reactions

Fortunately, allergic reactions to chemical peels are rare. As previously mentioned, resorcinol supposedly has the highest incidence of contact allergies. I am unaware of any reported allergies to TCA or glycolic acid. However, I have seen cholinergic uticaria triggered by TCA peeling (Fig. 10-13). It responded promptly to oral antihistamines, and I was able to block its occurrence on a second peel with prophylactic oral hydroxyzine (Atarax) administered 1 hour before the peel.

The problem with allergic reactions is that they can be difficult to diagnose. Because patients often have erythema and edema associated with the peel, these symptoms are not useful for diagnosing an allergic reaction. An allergy needs to be recognized and addressed promptly because skin undergoing an allergic reaction heals slower and with a greater risk of complication.

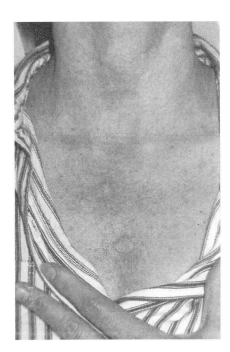

Figure 10-13
Urticarial papules on the neck and chest of a patient undergoing a level 2 TCA peel of the face. This patient had a history of cholinergic urticaria.

As a general rule, suspect an allergic reaction in the following situations:

▶ The patient has significant itching within a few hours of the peel (itching usually doesn't occur until a few days afterward)
▶ The patient has significant edema within a few hours of a light or medium depth peel (swelling is usually not pronounced until 24 to 48 hours after the peel and then usually only with peels of the papillary dermis or deeper)
▶ Erythema and edema are seen on the upper neck or in other areas that were not actually peeled
▶ Areas of urticaria (hives) appear on the body, or the patient has constriction in the throat with difficulty breathing (this is obviously a medical emergency and demands prompt treatment with epinephrine)

▷ Persistent Erythema

Some degree of erythema is common after almost any type of peel. Although some patients may initially have areas that are bright red, these usually fade into a light red or pink in 7 to 14 days. At 3 weeks after a peel, there normally are no areas of significant erythema. Areas that stay persistently red for more than 3 weeks are often a warning sign that an incipient scar may be forming in that location (Fig. 10-14). These areas usually are dusky red or red–purple rather than the bright red initially seen after a peel. If these areas are left untreated, they usually become indurated and progress into thickened, hypertrophic scars. Areas of persistent erythema 3 weeks after a peel should be viewed as definite precursors to scars and need to be treated aggressively.

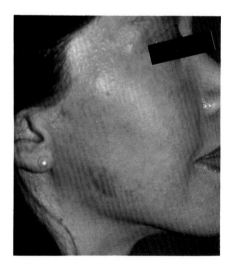

Figure 10-14

Area of persistent dusky erythema by the angle of the jaw weeks after a level 3 TCA peel.

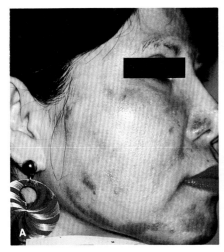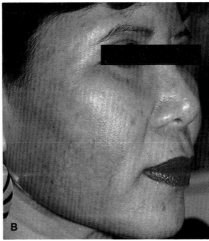

Figure 10-15
(*A*) Persistent erythema and induration 4 weeks after a TCA peel of unknown depth. (*B*) The same patient 3 weeks after applying clobetasol diporprionate cream (Temovate) twice a day to the areas of erythema. There is complete resolution of the erythema and induration.

The treatment modalities described below are basically the same as those for early hypertrophic scarring. The key here is to be aggressive, but not overly so. Intralesional steroids are not an appropriate therapy at this time, since they will induce atrophy in these patients. There are four possible treatments:

Class I ultrapotent topical corticosteroids (betamethasone [Diprolene], clobetasol [Temovate], halobetasol [Ultravate], diflorasone [Psorcon]): These are often capable of reversing persistent erythema in less than 2 weeks of use (Fig. 10-15). (See section on scarring.)

Steroid-impregnated tape: Cordran tape is a clear tape impregnated with a corticosteroid (flurandrenolide). The tape is applied to inflamed areas and left in place for 12 hours, then changed. It acts as an occlusive layer to enhance the penetration of the steroid while protecting the underlying tissue from further trauma. In most patients, the class I topical corticosteroids are far more effective than the steroid present in this tape. However, for patients who constantly rub or pick at their skin, the protection offered by the tape can be useful.

Silastic sheeting: These clear sheets are effective in reducing persistent erythema if they are worn continuously for a period of weeks to months. The major drawback is that they are unsightly to wear on the face and are difficult to tape in place there. (See section on scarring.)

Laser: The Candela pulsed dye laser can effectively reduce persistent erythema. It has two drawbacks:

- ▶ The treatment creates purpura that is rather unsightly for 1 to 3 weeks.
- ▶ The machine is expensive, so each treatment is more expensive than the other modalities mentioned here.

Whatever method you choose should be continued until the erythema resolves.

▷ Scarring

For most physicians and patients, the worst complication is scarring. Those at risk for scarring include the following:

- ▶ Patients with histories of poor healing and keloid formation
- ▶ Patients undergoing deep peels
- ▶ Patients undergoing second peels without allowing the skin to adequately heal from the first peel or from recent facial surgery
- ▶ Patients recently on isotretinoin (Accutane) therapy
- ▶ Patients who develop an infection during the peel

Several types of scars are possible complications from skin peeling:

- ▶ Hypopigmented, flat, sheetlike areas with a shiny surface and no induration

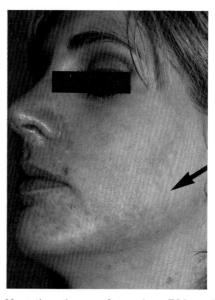

More than 1 year after a deep TCA peel

▶ Depressed atrophic areas often
with sharply demarcated, shelf-
like edges

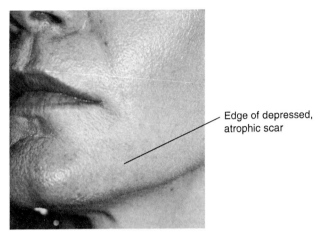

Edge of depressed,
atrophic scar

Six months after a deep TCA peel

▶ Thickened, elevated areas, often
with some degree of erythema

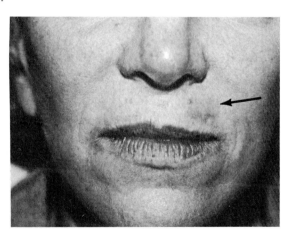

More than 1 year after a deep 50% TCA peel

▶ Severely hypopigmented or erythematous keloid-type scarring, which often causes tension deformities around the mouth or eyes (ectropion)

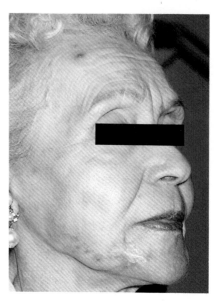

Several months after a deep TCA peel

Fortunately, scarring is an uncommon complication of chemical peeling. It appears to be directly related to the depth of the peel itself: the deeper the peel the greater the risk of scarring. Reticular dermal peels are far more apt to cause scarring than are papillary dermal peels. An uncomplicated intraepidermal peel should never create a scar.

Many cases of scarring are really secondary to another complication, such as infection, premature peeling, or trauma to the new tissue, rather than a direct complication of the chemical peel. Therefore, careful monitoring of the patient during the healing phase of the peel should allow you to identify and treat any of these predisposing factors before they lead to scarring.

During the past few years, a fair amount of evidence has suggested that patients who have previously taken isotretinoin (13-cis-retinoic acid) may have an increased tendency to develop scarring associated with dermabrasion or chemical peels performed after they have finished their isotretinoin therapy. The patients who have displayed this type of scarring have all had a similar type of atypical hypertrophic scar characterized by a stellate scar on the mid-cheek (an unusual location for a hypertrophic scar; Fig. 10-16). These atypical scars are associated with patients who had taken isotretinoin as long as 2 or 3 years before undergoing chemical peeling.

It would be prudent not to perform any peel for at least 1 year after a patient has completed use of isotretinoin. If the patient has had persistently dry skin since finishing isotretinoin therapy or has skin fragility, he or she should not undergo peeling with any agent (even the very superficial ones), until the skin has returned to its clinically normal pretreatment state, even if it means waiting 3 to 5 years.

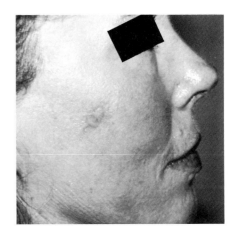

Figure 10-16

Atypical, somewhat stellate hypertrophic scar in a patient who underwent a level 3 TCA peel several months after completing a course of isotretinoin (Accutane).

The incidence of this type of scarring is extremely rare, but it has been reported in the literature so you must be aware of it. The exact mechanism of scar formation has not been determined. It may be secondary to decreased collagen remodeling due to decreased collagenase secondary to isotretinoin use.

Regardless of the cause, once scarring has begun to develop, it must be treated as rapidly and aggressively as possible. A mature scar is much more difficult to improve than a developing one. Flat or atrophic scars really don't respond well to any therapy. Fortunately, these are not as unsightly as the hypertrophic or keloidal scars, which are usually treatable.

At the first sign of persistent erythema or induration in any area after a peel, you should immediately begin treatment with either a class I ultrapotent topical corticosteroid cream applied twice a day or with some type of Silastic sheeting. Both these therapies have been highly successful in reversing erythema and induration and in preventing scar formation. It is far easier for most patients to use the topical corticosteroid twice a day than to wear a Silastic sheet taped to their skin for 24 hours a day. The sheet is unsightly (having a sheet of material taped to your face is an obvious cosmetic liability), but it is also difficult to tape into place during the first few weeks after a peel since the surrounding skin is sensitive and fragile at that time.

If you use one of the class I topical corticosteroids, it should be applied twice a day *only to the affected area*. Prolonged use of these products (more than 2 weeks) has been associated with steroid atrophy and the development of telangiectasias. Fortunately, indurated areas usually respond rapidly, within 1 week or so. In the case of induration and early scarring, it may take as long as 3 or 4 weeks to get complete resolution of the problem. I strongly believe it is worth the risk of steroid atrophy and telangiectasias to prevent scarring, particularly since telangiectasias can be treated with laser, and steroid atrophy can be treated with retinoic acid or AHAs.

Treatment of Scars

If, despite your best efforts, a problem area develops into true scar tissue you have several treatment options, as outlined below.

Silastic sheeting.   As previously discussed, Silastic sheeting can be effective but is not easy to use on the face. However, if a true scar has developed, the patient may be more highly motivated to wear the sheeting, particularly since it is the least aggressive therapy. Some people experience irritation or folliculitis from the sheeting, but most patients tolerate it well. This is a slow therapy, and both you and the patient need to be prepared to wait several months to achieve the best results.

Intralesional steroids.   These are probably the most commonly used therapy in the treatment of hypertrophic scarring. The most popular steroid to use is triamcinolone acetonide (Kenalog). The strength ranges from 1 to 40 mg/mL. When using intralesional steroids, there are several key points to keep in mind:

1. Inject the material directly into the scar, not into the surrounding tissue. Inadvertent placement of the steroid in the surrounding normal tissue will create atrophy and telangiectasias.
2. The injection works over a 2- to 3-week period. Any area of induration present at the end of that time needs to be retreated promptly or it will begin to grow and the scar will recur. The end point of intralesional therapy is a flat, supple area with no residual induration.
3. The concentration of the steroid needed is related to the thickness and maturity of the scar. Early, thin scars may respond to triamcinolone acetonide, 2 mg/mL, whereas thick older scars may need 30 to 40 mg/mL. However, it is usually best to start with 3 to 5 mg/mL for early scars and 10 mg/mL for thicker scars. It is important to increase the concentration of the steroid about 5 mg/mL with each successive injection if the scar is failing to respond.
4. Triamcinolone acetonide comes only in concentrations of 10 and 40 mg/mL. These liquids are actually a suspension of triamcinolone crystals rather than a solution. Therefore, they must be shaken thoroughly before being withdrawn from the bottle. The syringe should also be shaken before the injection to ensure uniform dispersion of the steroid particles. If the syringe is allowed to sit for 5 minutes, the particles will settle out of suspension, possibly inadvertently leading to too weak or too strong an injection.

   Also, when preparing a suspension in a different concentration than that supplied by the company (10 or 40 mg/mL), you need to dilute the original suspension with sterile water or saline. If you are attempting to create a suspension with a concentration below 10 mg/mL, always begin with the 10 mg/mL strength, not the 40 mg/mL strength.

The concentration of active steroid in each particle of 40 mg/mL is much greater than that found in the 10 mg/mL strength. Therefore, it is difficult if not impossible to create a suspension of 3 mg/mL by diluting the 40 mg/mL suspension. Attempting to do this will create a higher incidence of inadvertent overtreatment with resultant atrophy.

Scar excision and revision.   In patients prone to hypertrophic scarring and keloid formation, attempting to surgically excise a scar can be a risky proposition. The new surgical scar may hypertrophy, as happened with the original scar. However, if the scar was created by a secondary complication, such as infection or premature peeling, rather than the nature of how the patient heals from most wounds, there is an excellent chance for a successful revision.

Depending on the size and location of the scar, direct excision, Z-plasty, or even grafting may be considered as possible treatments. Because hypertrophic scars often improve spontaneously to a significant degree, it is prudent to **wait a minimum of 6 months after a peel before attempting to surgically revise a scar.**

Cryotherapy.   Some recent research has suggested that cryotherapy using liquid nitrogen can effectively treat hypertrophic scarring. Although this modality is an interesting "nonsurgical" therapy, it has a high incidence of creating hypopigmentation, an unacceptable complication on the face. Therefore, the usefulness of this procedure may be limited to nonfacial areas.

Radiation.   Although the popularity of radiation therapy for keloids and hypertrophic scarring has decreased, there may still be occasional times to consider this treatment.

Laser.   Some recent data presented by Goldman show that erythema and hypertrophic scarring can be markedly improved with the use of the Candela pulsed dye laser. Whether this is due only to an alteration and reduction of blood flow to the scar or some other direct effect on fibroblasts has yet to be elucidated. The possible risks with this therapy are minimal, so this treatment definitely deserves further research.

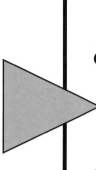

Manual of Chemical Peels: Superficial and Medium Depth, by Mark G. Rubin.
J.B. Lippincott Company, Philadelphia, © 1995.

CHAPTER 11

PATIENT SELECTION

Initial Consultation ▶ *Treatment Programs*

As physicians, most of us approach the idea of patient selection as a routine in which we attempt to fit the patient into a category of treatment based solely on the effectiveness of the therapy. This approach works well but doesn't give the patient much input into his or her therapy.

When treating photodamaged skin, several therapeutic options are available that offer a broad spectrum of levels of improvement, risk, and downtime. Therefore, it is important to offer the available treatment plan to patients and to allow them to choose the one that fits their life-style best. This information should be addressed during the initial consultation.

▷ Initial Consultation

With any cosmetic procedure, the most important step is the initial consultation. This really sets the stage for the physician–patient relationship and determines the patient's course of therapy. A poor consultation is really a set-up for problems later on. In this chapter, I will go over some general concepts of the interview and then discuss in detail parts of the consultation.

The purposes of the initial consultation are as follows:

▶ "Check out" each other's personality and establish a relationship
▶ Identify the patient's specific medical concerns
▶ Take a medical history that is sufficient to allow you to rule out patients with potential contraindications
▶ Evaluate the patient's acceptance of risk and downtime

▶ Educate the patient sufficiently to allow him or her to make an informed decision about treatment
▶ Set the ground rules for treatment

Establishing a Relationship

As physicians, we each have a certain style of practice and a specific approach to certain medical problems. Patients generally have a certain practice style that they prefer in their doctor as well. If you have an aggressive, abrupt domineering manner, and the patient prefers a chatty, low-key style, you may not "connect" well with the patient. If you don't interact well with him or her, it can make the goal of patient satisfaction more difficult to attain. It is important not to let a domineering patient take control of the consultation and direct you as to what procedures he or she thinks need to be done.

If your instincts tell you that something is wrong with performing a peel on a particular patient, listen to them. As clinicians, we develop a sixth sense about patients. Because peels are generally a cosmetic procedure, there is no reason that you can't easily and legally deny a patient a peel if you are not comfortable with the situation.

Identifying the Patient's Concerns

The first step in evaluating potential patients for chemical peels is to give them a mirror and have them show you exactly what they are unhappy with and want to improve. It is surprising how often what bothers patients is not what you initially notice when looking at their skin. So let the patients point out to you what brought them to your office, because it is extremely important that you understand and address these specific medical concerns of the patients first. Once you understand what they want to improve, you can point out any other skin conditions or lesions that can also be improved with the therapies you will be discussing.

Closely examining the skin (I usually use a 3× magnifying visor), both in a well-lit room and with a Wood's lamp, enables you to make an intelligent decision about the depth of peel needed.

Identifying Contraindications

With chemical peels, as with any procedure, certain patients are at greater risk for developing complications. In these cases, peels of certain depths may be contraindicated. You need to know this information before you arrange the patients' treatment plans.

Relative Contraindications

Inadequate sun protection: Any patients attempting to improve photo-damaged skin must prevent ongoing photodamage.

Pregnancy: Because the safety of peeling agents has not been examined in relation to pregnancy, medical and legal considerations suggest that peels not be performed on pregnant women.

Angina: Any peel capable of causing severe burning will elevate the pulse and blood pressure. Therefore, anything more than a very superficial peel should be avoided in patients with angina.

Recent head or neck injury: An area that has been wounded or undermined during recent surgery should not be peeled for a minimum of 2 to 3 months after operation.

History of radiation to the area to be peeled: Radiation causes atrophy of the pilosebaceous units, making reepithelialization more difficult. Therefore, only superficial peels should be done on areas of radiation damage, since they are prone to heal poorly. Never peel an area that has acute radiation injury.

History of keloidal scarring: It is safest to perform only intraepidermal peels on these patients or to avoid peeling them altogether.

History of herpes labialis: Patients with herpes can be peeled if they take oral acyclovir, but don't perform a peel over an actively infected area.

Open wounds or acne cysts in area to be peeled: Peeling over an open wound or inflamed acne lesion will intensify the depth of the peel in that area. It is best to avoid applying the peeling agent to these areas or to reschedule the peel.

Severe physical or mental stress: All peels are wounds of the skin. Patients need to be able to devote the appropriate time and energy to their healing process to achieve the best results.

Neurotic excoriation: Patients who constantly pick at their faces are at great risk of picking at their peeling skin, possibly inducing complications.

History of isotretinoin use within the past year: Evidence suggests that some patients who have taken isotretinoin (Accutane) 1 to 2 years before a dermal peel may have a higher incidence of atypical keloidal scarring.

In addition to these contraindications, both you and the patient should be aware that several conditions can be exacerbated by a chemical peel, including

- ▶ verruca plana
- ▶ herpes simplex
- ▶ seborrheic dermatitis
- ▶ atopic dermatitis
- ▶ perioral dermatitis
- ▶ acne rosacea
- ▶ facial telangiectasias

Evaluating the Patient's Acceptance
of Risk and Downtime

Once you have determined what needs to be treated, the next step is finding out what patients are willing to tolerate to get the results they desire.

Normally, after examining the patient's face, you will have decided how deep a peel is needed to provide the best results. Because there may be several treatment options, it is important to ask patients how aggressive a treatment regimen they want. This includes a discussion of possible therapies, their potential benefits, healing time (and impact on patient life-style), complications, and cost.

Educating the Patient

By discussing these options with patients, along with your recommendation, it allows them to make informed decisions about their treatment program. It also means that patients feel more responsible for their treatment, its benefits, and its downtime, since they chose it. In my practice, this has cut down significantly on patient complaints about healing time and its effect on work and social schedules. As an example, if a female patient presents with epidermal hyperpigmentation on the face, she has several treatment options:

a. A series of intraepidermal alpha hydroxy acid (AHA) peels. These have minimal or no downtime, but show slow, incremental improvement over several months.

b. A series of intraepidermal Jessner's peels. These produce more peeling than do AHA peels, but these patients usually can function almost normally. These patients often see more rapid improvement in their pigmentation than seen with AHA peels. This treatment program takes 6 to 8 weeks.

c. A full-thickness epidermal trichloroacetic acid (TCA) peel. This has about 5 days of downtime but offers the most dramatic improvement, so often only one treatment is needed.

In this situation, let the patient decide which treatment plan appeals most to her. If she chooses a series of AHA peels and is disappointed with the slow results, she can always move up to a more aggressive treatment plan. Such patients usually are not unhappy if this occurs because they knew from the start that they were doing the least aggressive therapy, with the slowest rate of improvement. If the patient chooses to undergo a full-thickness epidermal TCA peel and is frustrated with her appearance after 4 days of peeling, it is a simple and effective step to remind her that she chose the more aggressive therapy with more downtime in an effort to get the best results as rapidly as possible.

Allowing patients to choose their treatment program, rather than assigning them one, will save you more conflicts and unhappy patients than anything else you do.

Setting the Ground Rules

It is imperative that every patient follow your instructions exactly in order to give them the best results and the fewest complications. Some patients try to make deals with the doctor (eg, "After my TCA peel, can't I go into the tanning bed if I promise to stay in it only for 2 minutes?"). Many patients don't really believe that your rules or guidelines are made with their best interest in mind. If the patient doesn't want to follow your instructions or accept your recommendations in the initial consultation, this is someone you should not attempt to treat. I have found that patients who do not accept my rules in the beginning are often the ones who develop complications from peels later because they don't follow my instructions. Examples of this behavior include

> ▶ a patient with melasma who refuses to wear a broad-spectrum sunscreen because her makeup already contains a sunscreen with an SPF of 8
> ▶ a patient who refuses to believe your statement that one superficial AHA peel won't eliminate her deep wrinkles because she read in a women's magazine that it would
> ▶ a patient who you start on a regimen of retinoic acid and AHAs in preparation for a peel but who returns having used neither product, but rather a new European face cream her neighbor told her is the best thing for her skin

These examples may seem extreme, but I have seen these patients in my own office, and they are the same ones who develop complications with their peels because they use the wrong products on their skin, pick their peeling skin off, or go out in the sun too soon. And once patients develop complications, even if they created the problems, they will hold you responsible for them. So it is best to avoid this situation by terminating this relationship before even doing the peel. I routinely tell patients undergoing chemical peels that if they fail to follow my instructions, I will never peel them again because I will not be responsible for someone who won't follow directions. Most patients understand this type of approach and are then more inclined to follow instructions.

After reading this section, you may think it is written with an antagonistic slant, which was not my desire or intention. Actually, I think my office is very patient-oriented. However, having performed several thousand peels, I can tell you that strict adherence to the principles in this section will make both you and your patients happier. Remember, the goal of this section is to help you select the correct treatment for the correct patient (ie, to create the highest degree of patient satisfaction).

After the consultation you should have achieved several things:

GOALS OF THE INITIAL CONSULTATION

▶ An understanding of what you and the patient are attempting to correct on his or her skin
▶ An assessment of how deep the level of damage is on the patient's skin
▶ An appreciation of what the patient is willing to tolerate with respect to risk and downtime

---

▷ Treatment Programs

Integrating this information should make it easy to decide on the appropriate treatment plan. This is really the most important step in treating the patient. If you choose an inappropriate treatment plan, the patient will get suboptimal results.

The following few pages will illustrate, with the use of outlines, how your decision-making process should proceed.

Complaint: Rough-textured, dull-looking complexion

Due to: Thick stratum corneum

Therapy: Fortunately, this is very easy to treat, and anything you do will improve the skin.

Conservative (No Peeling)

It will take 3 to 6 weeks to achieve maximum improvement. The patient needs to thin the stratum corneum and to keep it thin to maintain the improvement. Treatment options are as follows:

a. Retinoic acid—This should not be used if patient has dry or sensitive skin, facial telangiectasias, or marked sun exposure.
b. AHA cream, lotion, or gel—This is well tolerated by most patients.
c. Salicylic acid cleanser—This has a tendency to be too drying in mature skin types.
d. Abrasive scrub—This has a tendency to be a bit drying and is often not effective enough.
e. Combinations of the above products

Aggressive (Peeling)

Skin will improve within days of the first peel, but more than one peel may be needed to achieve the best results. (Remember, patients need to be primed before the peel and kept on maintenance therapy afterward.) Peel options include the following:

a. 10% TCA—End point is level 0 frost; causes some shiny appearance to the skin and possible light exfoliation
b. Jessner's solution—End point is level 1 peel; similar healing appearance to that with TCA
c. 50% to 70% Glycolic acid—End point is mild erythema; usually creates no exfoliation
d. A single application of any of the above peeling agents with an end point the next level higher will give the patient an excellent result with only one treatment but will create more significant exfoliation and erythema.

Complaint: Epidermal melasma (hyperpigmentation)

Due to: Hormonal influence, genetics, sun exposure

Therapy: The goal of treating epidermal hyperpigmentation is to block the formation of new melanin with a tyrosinase inhibitor and to exfoliate the epidermis to decrease the amount of melanin present in the epidermis. If the hyperpigmentation developed while the patient was pregnant or taking birth control pills and she is no longer pregnant or off the pill, she usually will respond better than if her hormones are still "adulterated." If the patient developed melasma without any underlying cause, the response is variable, since the skin's current "steady state" is hyperpigmented. Your therapy does not change the skin's desire to return to that steady state, it only suppresses it.

Conservative

No downtime is associated with conservative treatment. Treatment is as follows:

a. 10% Glycolic acid with 2% to 4% hydroquinone, or 6% AHA with 2% kojic acid and 2% hydroquinone twice a day for 6 weeks with a broad-spectrum sunscreen applied every morning

If not better:

b. Addition of retinoic acid at bedtime if the skin can tolerate it
c. 50% to 70% Glycolic acid peels every 2 weeks—End point is mild erythema
d. Jessner's solution or superficial TCA peel every 2 weeks—Works faster than the glycolic acid peels but creates exfoliation

Aggressive

Patients must be on some type of bleaching agent and a broad-spectrum sunscreen before and after their peel (in addition to the medications for priming the skin). Peel options include the following:

a. Jessner's peels—End point is level 3 frost; causes heavy exfoliation and moderate erythema
b. 70% Glycolic acid—End point is patching epidermolysis; causes patching areas of erythema and crusting
c. 25% to 35% TCA—End point is level 2 frost; 5 to 6 days of dark skin and peeling; the most effective option in this category

Complaint: Epidermal postinflammatory hyperpigmentation

Due to: Reactive process to previous inflammation worsened by sun exposure

Therapy: The therapy of epidermal postinflammatory hyperpigmentation is the same as that for epidermal melasma. You need to block the production of new melanin and attempt to exfoliate the epidermis. You must be very careful that you **do not create inflammation with your treatment or it will induce more hyperpigmentation.** Therefore, there really are no safe aggressive therapies for postinflammatory hyperpigmentation, since any aggressive therapy will create erythema.

Conservative

1. If there is any evidence of inflammation, initially use a weak corticosteroid (class 6 or 7) twice daily, *then*
2. 10% glycolic acid with 2% to 4% hydroquinones, or 6% AHA with 2% kojic acid and 2% hydroquinone once or twice a day, depending on the patient's tolerance; use a broad-spectrum sunscreen every morning

If not better, the options are as follows:

a. Add retinoic acid at bedtime—Low level only; do not create inflammation
b. 50% Glycolic acid peels every 2 to 3 weeks if tolerated— End point is very mild erythema
c. Jessner's solution or superficial TCA peel every 2 to 3 weeks if tolerated—End point is very mild erythema

Aggressive

There are no aggressive treatments; all are too risky.

Complaint: Dermal hyperpigmentation

Due to: Melanin in the dermis (determined by Wood's light examination); includes dermal melasma and postinflammatory hyperpigmentation

Therapy: Dermal hyperpigmentation is difficult to treat.

 Topical bleaching agents may be slightly helpful, but they are not sufficient on their own.
▶ Papillary dermal peels give variable results.
▶ Reticular dermal peels can be quite effective (except for variable results with melasma), but they leave some residual hypopigmentation.

Complaint: Actinic keratoses

Due to: Atypical keratinocytes in the epidermis, possibly extending down the hair follicle; lesions are usually hyperkeratotic and thus more resistant to peels

Therapy: There are several potential therapies. Your ultimate goal is to destroy the abnormal cells, not just to make the skin feel smooth.

Conservative

With conservative treatment, it can take 6 to 12 months to achieve a good result. The keratosis may flare up with this therapy and appear worse for several months. Therapy options are as follows:

a. Retinoic acid in as high a strength as tolerated—Not for patients with sensitive skin, telangiectasias, or marked sun exposure
b. AHA in as high a strength as tolerated—Constantly try to increase the strength
c. Combination of retinoic acid and AHA
d. Salicylic acid cleanser—Helps remove the hyperkeratoses associated with actinic keratoses, enhancing the penetration of the other agents
e. Any of the above with the addition of 5-fluorouracil cream twice a day 1 or 2 days a week for pulse therapy

Aggressive (Peels)

Although repetitive superficial peels improve the clinical appearance of actinic keratoses, the lesions have a tendency to recur rapidly unless the patient stays on an aggressive regimen of home care products as discussed above. Many patients prefer the aggressive, one-shot-deal approach and don't want to stay on home care products. Therefore, I suggest these patients undergo papillary dermal peels to destroy as many of the keratoses as possible at one time. These patients benefit from prepeel 3- to 5-minute scrubs to reduce their hyperkeratoses. Treatment options are as follows:

a. 30% to 45% TCA (depending on the patient's skin type)—End point is level 3 frost; 5 to 8 days of downtime
b. 35% TCA with Jessner's solution, glycolic acid, or solid carbon dioxide—End point and downtime are similar to those with 30% to 45% TCA; you can specifically treat each lesion more aggressively with the first wounding agent to ensure better penetration of the TCA

Complaint: Fine wrinkles
Due to: Atrophy of the epidermis and dermis; *not due* to muscle movement
                 or gravitational effects
Therapy: A small percentage of these patients may achieve a miraculous
                 result with home care products, including retinoic acid and AHA.
                 However, most patients require more aggressive therapy.

Conservative

Options for therapy are as follows:

a. Retinoic acid at bedtime and an AHA product every morning—Since it appears
these two products have a synergistic effect, they should be used together.
b. Abrasive or salicylic acid cleanser—If the patient can tolerate 0.1% retinoic
acid cream at bedtime and a 15% to 20% AHA every morning without irritation,
try adding these cleansers to enhance the penetration of the retinoic acid and
AHA.
c. Series of 70% glycolic acid peels—Some patients can achieve excellent wrinkle reduction with multiple, very light glycolic acid peels with minimal or no
downtime.
d. Injectable collagen implants into the areas that fail to respond to the options
listed above.

Aggressive

These patients need to create epidermal thickening and more collagen and glycosaminoglycan deposition in the dermis to tighten their skin. I have been routinely
disappointed with repeated Jessner's peels and superficial TCA peels as therapy
for these patients. Treatment is as follows:

TCA or enhanced TCA peels—End point is level 3 frost in areas of wrinkling; 5 to 8
days of downtime

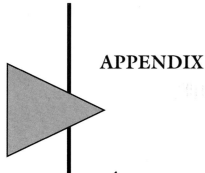

APPENDIX

AVAILABILITY OF PRODUCTS

Trichloracetic acid, Jessner's solution, salicylic acid ointment	Dermatologic Lab & Supply (800) 831-6273
Wood's light	Dermatologic Lab & Supply (800) 831-6273

Sunscreens

Shade UVA Guard	Schering Corporation (908) 298-4000
Ti-Screen (including chemical free)	T/I Pharmaceuticals (800) 782-0222
Neutrogena Moisturizer Sunscreen SPF 15 and Chemical-Free Sunblock	Neutrogena Dermatologic (213) 642-1150
Hawaiian Tropic Chemical-Free Sunscreen	Tanning Research Lab, Inc. (904) 677-9559
Dura-Screen (waterproof)	Penederm (800) 395-DERM
Shade 45 (waterproof)	Schering Corporation (908) 298-4000

Moisturizers

Eutra Products	Swiss-American Products, Inc. (800) 63Eutra
Moisturel	Westwood/Squibb (716) 887-3773
Complex 15 Moisturizer	Schering Corporation (908) 298-4000
DML Dermatological Moisturizing Lotion	Person & Covey, Inc. (800) 423-2341
Pen-kera	B.F. Ascher (913) 888-1880
Theraplex	Medicis Pharmaceuticals (800) 700-5866

Lightening Products

Eldoquin Forte 4% Bleaching Cream (4% hydroquinone cream)	ICN Pharmaceuticals (800) 548-5100
NeoStrata Lightening Gel (10% glycolic acid with 2% hydroquinone)	NeoStrata Company, Inc. (800) 628-9904
Azequin (11.7% azelaic acid)	Cardiovascular Research (415) 827-2636
Aza-Gel (15% azelaic acid)	Allergy Research Group (800) 545-9960
Melazepam (20% azelaic acid)	Strata Dermatologics (800) 888-4585/351-9429
Pigment Gel Phaze 13 (AHA blend with 2% hydroquinone and 2% kojic acid)	Physician's Choice of Arizona (800) 758-8185
Pigment Gel Forte (AHA blend with 2% hydroquinone and 4% kojic acid)	
Pigment Gel HQ Free (AHA blend with 3% kojic acid)	
Pigment Gel Forte HQ Free (AHA blend with 4% kojic acid)	

Postpeel Cortisones

Desowen Cream

Owen/Galderma Laboratories
(817) 293-0450

Locoid Cream

Ferndale Labs
(313) 548-0900

Aclovate Cream

Glaxo Dermatology Products
(800) 5GLAX05

Synalar Ointment

Syntex
(415) 855-5050

Antibiotic Ointments

Iobrom Gel

Physician's Choice of Arizona
(800) 758-8185

Bactroban Ointment

Beecham Laboratories
(800) BEECHAM

Garamycin Ointment
(pharmacy generic brand acceptable)

Schering Corporation
(908) 298-4000

Polysporin Ointment
(*never* use Neo-Sporin creams or ointments)

Burroughs Wellcome Co.
(919) 248-3000

Noncortisone Antiinflammatory

Catrix Cream

Donell, DerMedex
(800) 526-3461

Cortisones for Hypertrophic Scars

Temovate

Glaxo Dermatology Products
(800) 5GLAXO5

Ultravate

Westwood Squibb
(716) 887-3773

Diprolene

Schering Corporation
(908) 298-4000

Cordran Tape

Dista Products Co.
(317) 276-3714

**Silicone Occlusive Sheeting for
Hypertrophic Scars**

SIL-KS.F. Group Inc.
(800) 864-4386

CVI Corp.
(800) 872-4749

Biodermis
(800) 322-3729

Alpha Hydroxy Acids

Pyruvic acid

Lactic acid

Glycolic acid
(technical and reagent grade)
Glycolic acid 50% to 70% solutions

Sigma Chemical Company
(314) 771-5757

Spectrum Chemical Co.
(800) 772-8786

Dermatologic Lab & Supply
(800) 831-6273

Crown Drugs
(800) 85-CROWN

M.D. Formulations
(800) 633-6768

NeoStrata Company, Inc.
(800) 628-9904

Pharmagen Inc.
(800) 445-2595

Low-Dose Consumer Products

AHA Skin Smoothing Cream
(8%) glycolic acid)

AHA Skin Smoothing Lotion
(10% glycolic acid)

AHA Face Cream
(15% glycolic acid)

AHA Lotion
(15% glycolic acid)

AHA Solution for Oily and Acne-Prone
Skin
(8% glycolic acid)

NeoStrata Company, Inc.
(800) 628-9904

or

Dermatologic Cosmetic Laboratories
(800) 552-5060

AHA Gel for Age Spots and Skin Lightening
(10% glycolic acid, 2% hydroquinone)

AHA Enhanced Gel Formula
(15% glycolic acid)

Aqua Glyde Solution   Herald Pharmacal
(10% glycolic acid)   (800) 253-9499

Aqua Glycolic Face Cream
(10% glycolic acid)

Aqua Glycolic Lotion
(12% glycolic acid)

Glycare 5 Solution   M.D. Formulations
(5% glycolic acid)   (800) 633-6768

Glycare 10 Solution
(10% glycolic acid)

Facial Cleanser   M.D. Formulations
(10% glycolic acid)   (800) 633-6768

Facial Lotion
(10% glycolic acid)

Smoothing Complex   Veritas
(10% glycolic acid)   (602) 271-9577

Hand and Body Cream
(12% glycolic acid)

Lactic Acid Products

Lac-Hydrin 12   Westwood
(12% lactic acid)   (716) 887-3773

Penecare   Penederm
(5 and 7½ lactic acid)   (800) 395-DERM

Theraderm Skin Care System   Therapon
(lactic acid moisturizer, cleanser, and peel)   (501) 443-6632

AHA Blends

(lactic, citric, malic, tartaric; no glycolic)

Phaze 1–13 Skin Care System   Physician's Choice of Arizona
(AHA blend cleansers, moisturizers,   (800) 758-8185
toners, peel, etc.)

Azelaic Acid

Azequin 11.7%   Cardiovascular Research
                                               (415) 827-2636

Aza-Gel 15%   Allergy Research Group
                                               (800) 545-9960

Melazepam 20%   Strata Dermatologies
                                               (800) 888-4585/351-9429

Salicyclic Acid Cleansers

Sal Ac (2% salicyclic acid)   Genderm
                                               (800) 533-3376

Neutrogena Oil-Free Acne Wash   Neutrogena Dermatologic
                                               (213) 642-1150

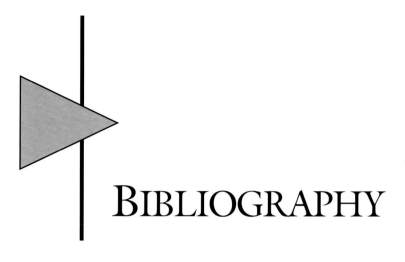

BIBLIOGRAPHY

GENERAL

Balin A, Pratt L. Physiological consequences of human skin aging. Cutis 1989;43:431–436.

Duffy DM. Informed consent for chemical peels and dermabrasion. Dermatol Clin 1989;7:183–185.

Goodson W, et al. Augmentation of some aspects of wound healing by a "skin respiratory factor." J Surg Res 1976;21:125–129.

Kaplan JZ. Acceleration of wound healing by a live yeast cell derivative. Arch Surg 1984;119:1005–1008.

Slue W. Photographic cures for dermatologic disorders. Arch Dermatol 1989;125:960–962.

Spira M, Freeman R, et al. Clinical comparison of chemical peeling, dermabrasion, and 5-FU for senile keratosis. Plast Reconstr Surg 1970;46:61–66.

Taylor C, et al. Photoaging/photodamage and photoprotection. J Am Acad Dermatol 1990;2:1–15.

AGING SKIN AND SKIN CLASSIFICATION

Fitzpatrick TB. The validity and practicality of sun-reactive skin types I through VI. Arch Dermatol 1988;124:6:869–871.

Ghersetich G, Grappone C, Dini G. Hyaluronic acid in cutaneous intrinsic aging. Int J Dermatol 1994;33:2:119–122.

Gilchrest B, et al. Chronologic and actinically induced aging in human facial skin. J Invest Dermatol. 1983;80:815–855.

Kligman AM, Lauker RM. Cutaneous aging: the difference between intrinsic aging and photoaging. J Cutan Aging Cosmet Dermatol 1988;1:5–11.

PIGMENTATION

Dreosti I, McGown M. Antioxidants and UV-induced genotoxicity. Res Comm Chem Pathol Pharmacol 1992;75:251–254.

Engasser P, Maibach H. Cosmetics and dermatology: bleaching creams. J Am Acad Dermatol 1981;5:143–147.

Gilchrest B, Fitzpatrick TB, et al. Localization of melanin pigmentation in the skin with Wood's lamp. Br J Dermatol 1977;96:245–248.

Kligman AM, Willis I. A new formula for depigmenting human skin. Arch Dermatol 1975;111:40–48.

Lotter AM. Human pigment factors relative to chemical face peeling. Ann Plast Surg 1979;3:231–240.

Mishima Y. Histopathology of functional pigmentary disorders. Cutis 1978;21:225–230.

Pathak M. Sunscreens and their use in the preventive treatment of sunlight induced skin damage. J Dermatol Surg Oncol 1987;13:739–750.

Pathak M, Fitzpatrick T, Kraus E. Usefulness of retinoic acid in the treatment of melasma. J Am Acad Dermatol 1986;15:894–899.

Pierce H, Brown L. Laminar dermal reticulotomy and chemical face peeling in the black patient. J Dermatol Surg Oncol 1986;12:69–73.

Stiller M, Davis I, Shupak J. A concise guide to topical sunscreens: state of the art. Int J Dermatol 1992;31:540–548.

Taylor C, et al. Photoaging, photodamage and photoprotection. J Am Acad Dermatol 1990;22:1–15.

Verallo-Rowell VM, et al. Double blind comparison of azalaic acid and hydroquinone in the treatment of melasma. Acta Dermatol Venereol 1989;143(Suppl):58–61.

NONPEEL THERAPIES

Marks R, Hills S, Barton SP. The effects of an abrasive agent on normal skin and on photodamaged skin in comparison with topical tretinoin. Br J Dermatol 1990;123:457.

Wilhelm K, Saunders J, Maibach H. Increased stratum corneum turnover induced by subclinical irritant dermatitis. Br J Dermatol 1990;122:793–798.

BASIC PEEL INFORMATION

Aronson RB. Hand chemosurgery. Am J Cosmet Surg 1984;1:24–28.

Ayres S III. Superficial chemosurgery in treating aging skin. Arch Dermatol 1962;85:125–133.

Ayres S III. Superficial chemosurgery, its current status and relationship to dermabrasion. Arch Dermatol 1964;89:395–403.

Baker TJ, Gordon HL. Chemical face peeling and dermabrasion. Surg Clin North Am 1971;51:387–401.

Brody H. Ethics in chemical peeling. J Dermatol Surg Oncol 1991;17:620–621.

Brody H. Letter to the editor. J Dermatol Surg Oncol 1991;17:622.

Collins PS. The chemical peel. Clin Dermatol 1987;5:57–74.

Collins PS, et al. Superficial repetitive chemosurgery of the hands. Am J Cosmet Surg 1984;1:22–24.

Epstein E, Epstein E, Jr. Skin surgery, ed 6. Philadelphia, WB Saunders, 1987:412–438.

Matatasso S, et al. The role of chemical peeling in the treatment of photodamaged skin. J Dermatol Surg Oncol 1990;16:945–954.

Matarasso S, Glogau R. Letter to the editor. J Dermatol Surg Oncol 1991;17:623–624.

Peikert JM. Exploring the efficacy of degreasing agents in the TCA peel. Cosmet Dermatol 1994;7:5:31–32.

Rubin M. Trichloroacetic acid and other non-phenol peels. Clin Plast Surg 1992;19:525–536.

Swinehart JM. Salicylic acid ointment peeling of the hands and forearms. J Dermatol Surg Oncol 1992;18:495–498.

Stegman S, Tromovitch TA. Cosmetic dermatologic surgery. Chicago, Year Book Medical Publishers, 1984:27–46.

Brody H, ed. J Dermatol Surg Oncol 1989;15a (entire issue).

RETINOIDS

Christopher EM, et al. A photonumeric scale for the assessment of cutaneous photodamage. Arch Dermatol 1992;128:347–351.

Ellis CN, et al. Sustained improvement with prolonged topical tretinoin (retinoic acid) for photoaged skin. J Am Acad Dermatol 1990;23:629–637.

Gardner S, Weiss J. Clinical features of photodamage and treatment with topical tretinoin. J Dermatol Surg Oncol 1990;16:925–931.

Goldfarb M, et al: Topical tretinoin and photoaged skin. Cutis 1989;43:476–482.

Griffiths CE, et al. Topical tretinoin treatment of hyperpigmented lesions associated withphotoaging in Chinese and Japanese patients: a vehicle-controlled trial. J Am Acad Dermatol 1994;30:76–84.

Hevia O, et al. Tretinoin accelerates healing after trichloroacetic acid chemical peels. Arch Dermatol 1991;127:678–682.

Hunt TK. Vitamin A and wound healing. J Am Acad Dermatol 1986;15:817–821.

Huong VC, et al. Topical tretinoin and epithelid wound healing. Arch Dermatol 1989;125:65–69.

Kligman AM, et al. Topical tretinoin for photoaged skin. J Am Acad Dermatol 1986;15:836–859.

Mandy S. Tretinoin in the preoperative and postoperative management of dermabrasion. J Am Acad Dermatol 1986;15:878–879.

Marks R, et al. The effects of an abrasive agent on normal skin and on photoaged skin in comparison with topical tretinoin. Br J Dermatol 1990;123:457–466.

Moy R, et al. Systemic isotretinoin: effects on dermal wound healing in a rabbit ear: model in vivo. J Dermatol Surg Oncol 1990;16:1142–1146.

Olsen EA, et al. Tretinoin emollient cream: a new therapy for photodamaged skin. J Am Acad Dermatol 1992;26:215–224.

Pinski KS. Isotretinoin patients may develop atypical scars following chemical peels on dermabrasions. Cosmet Dermatol 1992;5:41–42.

Pinski K, et al. Dermabrasion and retinoid therapy in dermatology today and tomorrow, vol 16. London, Mediscript, 1989.

Roenigk H, et al. Acne, retinoids and dermabrasion. J Dermatol Surg Oncol 1985;11:396–398.

Sendagorta ES, et al. Topical isotretinoin for photodamaged skin. J Am Acad Dermatol 1992;27:S15–S18.

Voorhees J, Orfanos C. Oral retinoids. Arch Dermatol 1981;117:418–421.

Weiss J, et al. Topical tretinoin improves photoaged skin. JAMA 1988;259:527–532.

ALPHA HYDROXY ACIDS

Ditre C, Van Scott E. Improvement of photodamaged skin with alpha hydroxy acids. Presented at the Update on Alpha Hydroxy Acid Symposium. San Diego, June 1993.

Elson M. The utilization of glycolic acid in photoaging. Cosmet Dermatol 1992;5:12–15.

Griffin T, Van Scott EJ. Use of pyruvic acid in the treatment of actinic keratoses: a clinical and histopathologic study. Cutis 1991;47:325–329.

Kligman A. Results of a pilot study evaluating the compatability of topical tretinoin in combination with glycolic acid. Cosmet Dermatol 1993;6:10:28–32.

Lavker RM, Kaidbey K, Leyden J. Effects of topical ammonium lactate on cutaneous atrophy from a potent topical corticosteroid. J Am Acad Dermatol 1992;26:535–544.

Moy LS. A comparison of depths of wounding of different peeling agents. Presented at the Update on Alpha Hydroxy Acid Symposium. San Diego, June 1993.

Piacquadio D, Grove M, Dobry M. Efficacy of glycolic acid peels questioned for photodamaged skin. Dermatol Times, May 1992.

Van Scott EJ. The unfolding therapeutic uses of the alpha hydroxy acids. Mediguide Dermatol 1988;3:1–5.

Van Scott EJ, Yu RJ. Hyperkeratinization, corneosyte cohesion and alpha hydroxy acids. J Am Acad Dermatol 1984;11:867–879.

Van Scott EJ, Yu RJ. Alpha hydroxy acids: procedures for use in clinical practice. Cutis 1989;43:222–228.

TRICHLOROACETIC ACID

Brodland D, Roenigk R. Trichloroacetic acid chemex foliation (chemical peel) for extensive premalignant actinic damage of the face and scalp. Mayo Clin Proc 1988;63:887–896.

Brody H, Hailey C. Medium depth chemical peeling of the skin: a variation of superficial chemosurgery. J Dermatol Surg Oncol 1986;12:1268–1275.

Resnik SS. Chemical peeling with trichloroacetic acid. J Dermatol Surg Oncol 1986;10:549–550.

Resnik SS, Lewis LA. The cosmetic uses of trichloroacetic acid peeling in dermatology. South Med J 1973;66:225–227.

Resnik SS, Lewis LA, Cohen BH. Trichloroacetic acid peeling. Cutis 1976;17:127–129.

Roberts HL. The chloroacetic acids: a biochemical study. Br J Dermatol Syp 1926;38:323–334, 375–391.

Stegman S. Medium depth chemical peeling: digging beneath the surface. J Dermatol Surg Oncol 1986;12:1245–1246.

COMBINATION PEELS

Brody HJ, Chenault WH. Medium-depth chemical peeling of the skin: a variation of superficial chemosurgery. J Dermatol Surg Oncol 1986;12:1268–1275.

Coleman WP, Futrell IM. The glycolic acid–trichloroacetic acid peel. J Dermatol Surg Oncol 1994;20:76–80.

Monheit GD. The Jessner's and TCA peel: a medium depth chemical peel. J Dermatol Surg Oncol 1989;15:945–950.

Moy LS. Jessner's solution and 70% glycolic acid combination peels. Presented at AAD Annual Meeting. Washington DC, 1993.

HISTOLOGY

Ayres S III. Dermal changes following application of chemical cauterants to aging skin: superficial chemosurgery. Arch Dermatol 1960;82:578.

Baker TJ, Gordon HL, Mosienko P, Seckinger DL. Long-term histological study of skin after chemical face peeling. Plast Reconstr Surg 1974;53:522.

Behin F, Fuerstein AA, Marovitz WF. Comparative histological study of many pig skins after chemical peel and dermabrasion. Arch Otolargyngol 1977;103:271–277.

Brodland DG, Cullimore KC, Roenigk RK, Gibson LE. Depths of chemexfoliation induced by various concentrations and application techniques of trichloroacetic acid in a porcine model. J Dermatol Surg Oncol 1989;15:967–971.

Brody HJ. Variations and comparisons in medium-depth chemical peeling. J Dermatol Surg Oncol 1989;15:953–963.

Kligman AM, Baker TJ, Gordon HL. Long-term histologic follow-up of phenol face peels. Plast Reconstr Surg 1985;75:652–659.

Smith L. Histopathologic characteristics and ultrastructure of aging skin. Cutis 1989;43:414–424.

Spira M, Dahl C, Freeman R, Gerow FJ, Hardy SB. Chemosurgery: a histological study. Plast Reconstr Surg 1970;45:247.

Stegman SJ. A study of dermabrasion and chemical peels in an animal model. J Dermatol Surg Oncol 1980;6:490–497.

Stegman SJ. A comparative histologic study of the effects of three peeling agents and dermabrasion on normal and sun damaged skin. Anaesth Plast Surg 1982;6:123–135.

WOUND HEALING

Eaglestein WH, Mertz PM. "Inert" vehicles do affect wound healing. J Invest Dermatol 1980;47:90–91.

Elson ML. Effects of petroleum jelly on the healing of the skin following cosmetic surgical procedures. Cosmet Dermatol 1993;6:18–22.

Geronemur RG, Mentz PM, Eaglestein WH. The effects of topical antimicrobial agents. Arch Dermatol 1980;115:1311.

Gette MT, Marks JG, Maloney ME. Frequency of postoperative allergic contact dermatitis to topical antibiotics. Arch Dermotol 1992;128:365–367.

Hunter D, Frumkin A. Adverse reactions to vitamin E and aloe vera preparations after dermabrasion and chemical peel. Cutis 1991;47:193–196.

Peikert JM. Exploring the efficacy of degreasing agents in the TCA peel. Cosmet Dermatol 1994;7:5:31–32.

Rubin MG. The anti-inflammatory and wound healing effects of 20% Catrix ointment on TCA 35% peels. Presented at the American Society of Dermatologic Surgery Annual Meeting, Scottsdale, AZ, March, 1992.

Stuzin JM, Baker TJ, Gordon HL. Chemical peel: a change in the routine. Ann Plast Surg 1989;23:166–169.

COMPLICATIONS

Litton C, Trinidad G. Complications of chemical face peeling as evaluated by a questionnaire. Plast Reconstr Surg 1981;67:738–744.

Goldman M, Fitzpatrick R. The use of the candela pulsed dye laser in the treatment of hypertrophic scars. Presented at the American Academy of Dermatology Annual Meeting, Washington, DC, December 1993.

Pascher F. Systemic reactions to topically applied drugs. Bull NY Acad Med 1973;49:613–617.

Ross R. Problems in aesthetic surgery. St Louis, CV Mosby, 1986:339–373.

Spira M, Gerow FJ, Hardy SB. Complications of chemical face peeling. Plast Reconstr Surg 1974;54:397–403.

Stagnone G, Orgel M, Stagnone J. Cardiovascular effects of topical 50% trichloroacetic acid and Baker's phenol solution. J Dermatol Surg Oncol 1987;13:999–1002.

INDEX

Page numbers followed by *f* indicate figures; those followed by *t* indicate tables.

177